KERI
My Inspiration

Clodagh Sweeney

With love,

Clodagh
xxx

© 2024 Clodagh Sweeney 978-1-915502-54-4

All rights reserved. This book is a memoir and tribute to Keri written by the author, Keri's mother, on her recollections of events and experiences over time. The information presented is the author's opinion, backed up with legal and medical evidence where applicable and does not constitute any health or medical advice for another.

The content of this book is for informational purposes only and is not intended to diagnose, treat, cure, or prevent any condition or disease. The author and publisher attempt to ensure the accuracy of the information presented, however the information may contain some unintentional errors which they reserve the right to amend at any time and not be held liable for.

No part of this book may be reproduced, stored in a retrieval system, or transmitted by any means, electronic, mechanical, photocopying, recording or otherwise without written permission from the author. Published in Ireland by Orla Kelly Publishing. Cover image and other images used by the author.

Orla Kelly Publishing
27 Kilbrody,
Mount Oval,
Rochestown,
Cork,
Ireland.

*For Keri, Lucy and Mark,
you are my universe.*

Stargazer

The pain when
you came then
almost didn't
I drew strength from an oak
that swayed through the pane,
waving at me
in my crisis and crying,
I breathed its calm,
moving me in harmony
like the chord that
connected you and I
I was afraid

But you? You were just busy
turning your head
getting ready to see the
stars, not wanting to miss
the unveiling universe when
you, my love, were the
greatest reveal of all
I gave you life, but because
of you, I live it

© Imelda May 'A Lick And
A Promise' (Faber Music 2021)

Contents

1. Deal 1
2. Screaming 11
3. Dismissal 17
4. Pathways 23
5. Roly Poly... 36
6. Smiles... 45
7. Preschooler... 52
8. Sisterhood 58
9. Truth 68
10. Contentment... 73
11. Admission 77
12. Vindication 81
13. Neighbourhood 91
14. Spasms 97
15. Planning... 104
16. Separation 108
17. Mass.. 116
18. Romance 122
19. Curvature 129
20. The Dance.. 154
21. Santa 158

22. Athlete	161
23. Tenacity	168
24. London	179
25. Balance	195
26. Prognosis	202
27. Togetherness	206
28. Belle	213
29. VIP	225
30. Nuptials	230
31. Wings	235
32. Flight	241
33. Release	253
34. Healing	265
Words of Appreciation	273
Please Review	278

1

Deal

It is often said that our children choose us as their parents before they come into this world. What was it that Keri saw in me to make me the luckiest of all to have her as my girl? What did she see in that ordinary girl, in that ordinary life? Was there another layer to me that she could see that I knew nothing of?

When Keri danced from the stars to my belly in early 2003, I was married to Brendan, or Chalkie, as he is known. We met at a disco in 1994 when I was 19 years old and later worked together at Dawn Fresh Foods in Fethard. Chalkie was a line worker, and I was a receptionist. It was a fun time. After dating for a number of years, we committed to each other, building our bungalow together in Fethard, Co Tipperary, in 1997 when I was 21, and marrying in 1999 when I was 23. We enjoyed a few fantastic years, all the while optimistically planning for future family life. I was a happy-go-lucky girl. I had the honour of being appointed bridesmaid for my best friend, Noelle. Life was good.

The year 2002 was a big one for me, a year of beginnings and endings. It was the year when my beloved Daddy, Billy, a builder, died soon after being diagnosed with cancer, leaving behind my mother, Freddie, my three sisters Carmel, Fionnuala and Colette, my brother Liam and I. Daddy was taken too soon; we all still feel it. Mammy is strong. She has weathered that and many more storms since, but she rightly should still have him by her side.

It was also the year when I stepped out of secretarial roles and established a sandwich bar in Thurles, Co Tipperary, with my sister Carmel. She was a silent partner; I was in front of the house. I was invigorated running my own business; a lot of work, but I always thrived on working hard. It was building a financial foundation for the healthy, happy future family life that Chalkie and I planned for. I met one of my very best friends in life, Sharon, whilst working in the sandwich bar.

I never met my first baby, but I believe in my heart that he was a little boy, and his name is Billy. I had been pregnant for 14 weeks and had suffered cramps before we left for a week's holiday with friends in Turkey. The pain got progressively worse as the week went on, and what started as mild spotting soon progressed to heavy bleeding. I went to a doctor who gave me medication and was told to keep my legs elevated on the flight home. The following day, I became very unwell on the journey home. An ambulance collected me from Dublin airport, and I was taken to the Rotunda Maternity Hospital. Various tests were carried out, and I was told that I was losing my baby. There was nothing that could be done. I was sent home, but the pain didn't abate. I ultimately ended up in St Luke's Hospital in Kilkenny, where I went into full blown labour.

I suspect my baby fell away from me as I used the toilet during this time. I vividly remember hearing the drop into the toilet bowl. This moment sounded like the end of the physical pain and the end of my first pregnancy, but only the beginning of the feeling of emptiness and heartbreak that would leave Chalkie and I utterly devastated.

I fell pregnant with Keri in early 2003. She was very much planned and longed for. It was a healthy pregnancy. I felt physically great but emotionally apprehensive, given our prior loss. Keri was a healthy and active baby in the womb. My best friend Noelle was also expecting, 4 weeks after me, so we rode the waves of apprehension and excitement together. It was a special time. Scans confirmed a normal, healthy pregnancy. No abnormalities were found at any stage. Keri was developing perfectly.

I registered myself under the care of St Luke's Hospital, Kilkenny, where my nieces and nephews had been delivered. During an antenatal visit in the latter part of the pregnancy, I recall being asked about my shoe size in the context of my ability to give birth vaginally, which I found strange at the time. I am a small person, standing at just 5ft. I still don't know the medical relevance or credibility of this data, but the fact that I am a tiny shoe size 4 haunted me as I laboured, laboured, and laboured some more on the 19th and 20th of October 2003.

The earlier stages of the labour had been manageable; I was under the care of an incredibly kind and experienced Midwife. After the first labour-inducing gel was inserted, I walked the corridors of the hospital and waited for things to happen. Pains started to slowly develop as the day went on.

Staff changeover happened at 8pm, and a new Midwife came on duty. From then on, the atmosphere in my birthing room was entirely different. By then, I was measuring around 4cm dilated. A second gel was inserted to further progress my labour. As I had been complaining of constipation, I was given an enema. This resulted in a sudden, massive, painful bowel motion, after which I progressed immediately to 10cm dilation in agonising pain.

I begged for pain relief over and over again. I tried my best to be respectful. I was apologetic. I felt embarrassed and self-conscious. I wanted to keep my dignity. I didn't want to be shouting and screaming. I wanted to do as I was told and for the experts to look after me.

The brakes on the bed were lifted, and I was wheeled away from the gas and air on the wall, told I wasn't having it anymore. An epidural was not organised for me despite my ongoing pleas. I was told I was being impossible. I was repeatedly reminded that I was not the only patient in the hospital. Hours passed.

I just wanted my baby. I wanted us to be a family. I felt like I was submerged and drowning in a sea of confusion and incompetence.

A vacuum was taken out. I instinctively sensed immense danger. This was my first round of advocacy for my baby (there would be many more). Being the nice, quiet lady simply wasn't going to save my baby. I screamed at the Midwife that I would drive her through the walls with my feet if she came near me with the vacuum in her hands. I was terrified my baby would die.

A doctor came into the room, searching for something in a cabinet. I asked, 'Are you going to give it to me?' He didn't know what I was talking about. I told him I needed an epidural. He came over to my bedside and looked at the monitor. The Midwife was shouting that I was to be vacuumed but that I wouldn't let her do it. Eventually, she was silenced. The doctor looked at the monitor with a worried gaze. He asked me what I wanted. 'Get it out of me', I pleaded. At long last, the courtesy of being heard. He called for a caesarean and my nail varnish on my toes to be removed immediately.

Eventually, I was moved to a corridor outside the operating theatre, and a small team descended upon me. Some new faces, now-worried expressions, silent glances that terrified me. Still no pain relief. I was restrained while a catheter was agonisingly inserted as I pushed. A doctor called for everyone to stop, to leave me alone until I was put to sleep. Mercy at last. A 'crash' caesarean section was carried out. The cord was wrapped and tangled tightly around Keri's neck. She was asphyxiated.

The delivery was too late to save her from catastrophic brain damage, but timely enough that, equipped with her fierce little lion heart, my baby would fight and survive.

Groggy but awake, Chalkie announced that our baby was a girl. He was previously told that we had a boy, but then he learned that this was a mistake. He was also told that the baby was perfectly healthy. We were soon to learn that was, tragically, not so.

I fell back asleep. In and out of consciousness, asking about my baby each time I woke. I had been very heavily medicated, and it took some time to fully come around. All appeared well. Chalkie was told there was no problem. I rested my eyes. Our baby was fine, and the torment was over. This, too, was untrue.

A Paediatrician visited us in the morning. Out of the blue, we were told that our baby was critically ill and likely to die. We were flabbergasted. I felt absolute dismay. How could it be that our baby delivered the night before was so unwell, and yet nobody had told us? At that moment, I didn't believe her. For me, unless I see it, I don't believe it. We were asked if we would like her to be baptised. I requested that Father Breen (a beloved family friend who was in my life since childhood) be asked to come up from Fethard. That was not possible, we were told. This was too urgent. The hospital chaplain obliged. From our two favourites, Chalkie chose the name Keri over Shauna for our beautiful baby girl. It fitted her perfect little face. I was transported by a wheelchair to the neonatal unit for the baptism. Chalkie, my brother Liam and his wife Pamela also attended. The moment I laid eyes on my perfect little girl that morning, I fell instantly in love. She changed me that day. My heart became of her, and it beat for her: determined, resilient and overflowing with endless love. That has never changed.

I burst into tears. Keri was rigged up to wires, lines and tubes. I knew at that moment that we were in the worst nightmare and that this was real. Our precious little princess could very well die. I felt so helpless. I wasn't allowed to be close to her or to touch her, never mind fix her, which was all I wanted to do. A hug can fix so much, but not this time. While the quick baptism took place, a medical team stood by closely on the sidelines, carefully observing, ready to pounce on Keri should the various machines erupt. It was a fast baptism, over in a flash. A machine sounded, and we were asked to quickly leave.

I later learned that they lost Keri a couple of times during those initial hours. A neonatal squad came from Waterford Regional Hospital to Kilkenny to stabilise Keri, and they worked on her for many hours. (I also learned, years later, that it was some hours before Keri was properly intubated).

This was an exceptionally critical time. Keri suffered seizures and early but clear signs of multi-organ damage.

We were given very little hope that she would survive. We were told to prepare ourselves for her to die.

I repeated my side of the deal with God.

Let her live. I will look after the rest.

Keri and I became lioness and cub, fighting together for survival in the wilderness of a broken system, the perilous jungle that is the Irish Health Service Executive.

Baptised and stabilised, Keri was eventually deemed stable enough to transfer to Waterford Regional Hospital for ongoing intervention and care in their neonatal unit. Keri travelled by ambulance with a neonatal team who kept her stable for the journey. Chalkie and Liam travelled behind by car, and my ambulance followed, accompanied by Chaklie's mother, Mary. I didn't know why my baby was so sick, nor what would happen next. We raced through the streets, and my heart raced in terror.

I pleaded with God once again. *Let her live. Nothing else matters.*

I was admitted to a ward at Waterford Regional Hospital with pregnant women, mothers and babies. I cried and cried and cried behind my cubicle curtains. It was mere hours after my caesarean section, and my wound was oozing, making a mess of the sheets. I was ashamed of what was coming from my body and embarrassed that I had to be helped when really everyone should have been helping Keri alone. Tears of utter despair and devastation gushed from the pit of my stomach, bursting out in gasps and sobs. It was a huge mercy to be moved to a different floor the following day, where I was in a ward with another mother whose baby was also in the neonatal unit. We helped and supported each other as we expressed milk together for our sick babies.

Eventually, I was brought to see Keri again in her new hospital ward, only a tender few hours old. I watched as her little belly rose and fell with the ventilator. I was told that she was suffering seizures and that they were giving her phenobarbitone to control them. The staff were incredibly reassuring and gentle as they worked so hard to support Keri in her earliest battle to survive.

I urged my little angel: *Fight, don't go.* I knew at that moment that I needed her more than she would ever need me. That truth stands to this day.

During those initial days of Keri's life in intensive care at Waterford Regional Hospital, we began to learn what had happened to our baby. Chalkie and I were informed by a Paediatrician of a brain scan which had been taken, showing significant white matter damage.

I expressed breast milk for Keri; I was told it would really help her. She was fed by tube over the following weeks before being gradually weaned from the support machines and moved to the step-down neonatal unit. Slowly but surely, the seizure activity settled with medication. There was so much I didn't know. So much uncertainty. Once again, I told myself that as long as she was alive, we would be alright. I couldn't look beyond that.

It was time for action and to move ahead with this new life. A life more complex and more challenging, but a life with Keri, which was all I had asked for in that labour ward. She was all I needed. I swallowed the painkillers and got out of my hospital bed as quickly as I could. I requested discharge. I just couldn't pull myself together and be strong for Keri if I was walking around a hospital ward in pyjamas all day.

I put my game face on. I got myself moving to get my body and my head into the right space. With a face of makeup and proper clean clothes on, I was ready for the road ahead. Keri was suffering enough without me feeling sorry for myself. After a strong coffee, I put one foot in front of the other. My life wasn't about me anymore. I was going to keep my side of the deal. Keri was still very poorly. Nobody could say what would happen. I decided we would live every day like it was our last together. That became our way of life.

2

Screaming

I will never forget Keri's first journey home from hospital at three weeks of age. We were handed a cocktail of medication and sent on our way. As we drove home to Fethard, Keri screamed the entire journey. Chalkie and I were terrified.

The crying and distress continued unabated, such that, later that night, we ended up bringing her back to Waterford Regional Hospital. Keri was given further medication, and we were sent home again the following day.

Following our second homecoming, the screaming and crying persisted. Episode after episode, without reprieve or relief, Keri's tiny body would stiffen up as she held her breath until she went purple, followed by a violent and terrifying shake of her whole body. This cycle would loop, time and again, until she would collapse, exhausted, for a short few minutes of sleep. The cruel screaming and shaking loop would then commence all over again.

Keri suffered such torture in those early weeks. Little could be done by her medical team to relieve her pain, as she screamed for 18 to 20 hours a day. She cried so much that there were no tears. She was on *epilim* and *phenobarbitone* for her seizures, which we gave to her orally with a syringe. What we did to try and feed Keri during this time was simply barbaric. Keri was not able to latch onto the bottle. She was too distressed and, as it transpired, didn't have the oral-motor skills or the suck reflex to do so. We didn't understand any of this, nor was it ever explained to us. We kept trying to feed her, hour after hour. The only way we could do this was to squirt milk into her mouth as she screamed. We used a syringe to do this, to get the milk right back to her throat. Even with this, she barely took in any milk at all. Not only was she traumatised from her birth and in severe pain, but she was also famished. She lost a lot of weight.

By that point, Chalkie had gone back to work. As Chalkie was working with knives as a butcher, I was terrified he would suffer exhaustion and hurt himself, so I didn't ask for help overnight. It was essential that we had an income. I certainly could not leave Keri to go to work in the state she was in, so I insisted that he sleep.

Keri and I were alone at home while Chalkie worked to keep a roof over our heads. Keri would occasionally sleep for short bursts between crying episodes, but only on my chest. If I let her down to lie horizontally, she would immediately scream. The sofa became my bed as I sat up with her, day and night. The only place she was in any way comforted was in my arms.

I slept in short bursts, sitting up on the couch when I could. I didn't dare move in case I woke her exhausted little body. In those early days, over 24 hours, Keri and I got 3 to 4 hours sleep at most. I got the sense she had reflux, which was causing so much of her pain and distress, particularly around feeding. While it wasn't prescribed, I started Keri on *Losec,* which I managed to get my hands on. I knew all about the medical uses for it, having seen a family member do very well on it. After some persuading, I eventually got a prescription for it. I wasn't taking no for an answer.

Noelle delivered a beautiful, perfectly healthy baby boy, Keenan, exactly a month after Keri's birth. Noelle visited regularly, sitting with Keenan, Keri and I for hours, keeping us company, making sure I knew we were not alone in our despair. Despite the incessant screaming from Keri, Noelle never flinched. She never made the commonplace excuse that she had somewhere else to be when things got difficult or uncomfortable. She always stayed right by my side. Noelle is a lot taller than I am. Her hugs are firm, embracing and nourishing. Her personality is straight up, steady, honest, and incredibly kind. The developmental differences between Keri and Keenan were stark, but they never caused me distress. I enjoyed getting to know Keenan and watching him grow, genuinely delighted for Noelle that it had all worked out for her. Noelle's support and friendship held me up when I felt I could no longer stand.

I kept my game face on. Despite the anguish of Keri's condition, I was utterly in love. There was nowhere else I wanted to be than with her, soothing her, loving her. She needed me to be strong. I incrementally recalled my pact with God, shook myself down, put my chin up, renewed the game face and made another large mug of coffee.

During these initial months, Keri was in a desperately bad way. She remained so unsettled, in so much pain, unable to relax, unable to feed. We visited the GP clinic umpteen times during this period, and while we were met with so much compassion and concern, there was little that could be done for her medically.

At three months old, Keri was referred back to the hospital by her GP due to ongoing screaming up to 23 hours a day. She was admitted to the paediatric ward. To my dismay, I was addressed as follows; 'Now, Mrs Brett, I may as well be honest with you. Your daughter will never be anything, and she will never do anything. She will be a burden to you for the rest of your life. My advice to you is, you are a young woman, go off and have a proper family for yourself and forget you ever had her'. I asked what he meant by that, dismayed with what I heard so far. 'You don't need to worry. All you have to do is walk out those two doors right now, and we will look after the rest'. I saw red. I looked at him squarely, stood up from my chair and said 'my child is my flesh and blood. How dare you speak about her like that, who do you think you are?' He responded, 'There is nothing wrong with your child, only that she is a spoiled brat. You have her the way she is'. My last words to him were, 'Get out of this room before I stick you to the wall with a slap'. He responded, 'If you don't want to face facts, that is fine,' and he walked out. I have never hit anyone in my life, but I certainly did mean that. Within five minutes, I was scolded by another staff member for speaking with a senior doctor in such a fashion. I told her to get out of the room, too, or I would stick her to the other wall.

I stayed with her every moment of that time in the hospital for that week. I couldn't trust the system. I was so disillusioned. I had to protect Keri and advocate for her. The crying and feeding difficulties persisted. There was no reprieve.

I had to find another way.

I searched online for alternative or complementary therapies that might help Keri. It was Cranial Osteopathy that resonated most with me in terms of what Keri needed. Cranial Osteopathy is a very holistic approach, where gentle massage and manipulation of the head work to remove tensions which remain since the pregnancy/delivery. The aim is to restore balance, alignment in the body and wellbeing. That sounded like exactly what Keri needed after what she had been through. There was no doubt whatsoever that she didn't only have tension in her head, but her entire little body was in shock and misalignment.

I made an appointment with Ian Wright, a Cranial Osteopath in Clonmel, to see if he could help Keri. What started as one experimental session turned into a lifelong commitment by Ian to help Keri. Ian started by working on her head, where she needed help most. Ian's treatments provided great comfort for Keri, and I could see she was benefiting from them. Combined with mainstream medicine, alternative treatments like Osteopathy became our lifeline to a more comfortable life for Keri.

3

Dismissal

There were so many questions whirling in my mind about what had taken place at the hospital during Keri's birth. Chalkie and I requested a meeting with hospital management so that we could understand what had gone so desperately wrong. By the time this meeting took place, Keri was about 8 weeks old. She had screamed in pain for 20 of every 24 hours of her day up to that point. We had not received any support or follow up from St Luke's whatsoever. We were petrified and exhausted. We didn't know where or how things would ever improve for her.

When Chalkie and I attended, we met with a number of key management personnel. I was clear that I wanted an explanation and an apology for what happened before, during and after Keri's birth. Keri's life was irrevocably changed from the moment she was born. The brutality of what had happened to us simply could not happen to another family. Keri had survived, and I was overwhelmingly grateful for that. I would make it work, but they had to admit wrong was done. They had to say sorry to my little princess. This was the least she deserved. We were none the wiser leaving that first meeting. We were assured that things would be looked into, and another meeting was arranged in due course.

Some weeks later, we were summoned to return to St Luke's for a follow up. There was no information, clarification, or apology. I asked to meet the second Midwife who had presided over the later part of my labour. While initially that seemed possible, it was soon shut down by further echelons of management as an unreasonable request which might have negative consequences for the staff member involved. Our feelings and the negative consequences for Keri didn't seem relevant! To my utter disbelief, without apology, explanation, or offer of support, we were told in no uncertain terms that we should just go ahead and sue the hospital. My parting words were, 'If you want to play hardball, we will play hardball'. We were dismissed from the meeting. I made an appointment to see Cantillon's Solicitors without delay. My little girl was going to get her truth and her apology. I was not going to rest until that happened.

We told our story, and Ernest Cantillon and his assistant, Liz O Brien, listened carefully. The legal advice was daunting. The first question to be addressed was what should or should not have happened in managing my labour. Or what happened that shouldn't have? These are questions of negligence. To investigate them, we had to order and pay for multiple medicolegal reports from overseas experts in obstetrics and midwifery. Doctors in Ireland won't critique their friends' and colleagues' work in Court. The second question was causation. If negligence were confirmed, further expensive reports would be required to confirm that it, and nothing else, caused Keri's brain damage. Such experts would include Paediatricians, Paediatric Neurologists and Neuroradiologists, who would examine patterns of her condition, both clinically and on a brain scan, to establish if she was injured from the negligence or if it was, in fact, an unrelated, natural cause.

We were advised that if the reports went against the case, we would leave with nothing. There is no legal aid in Ireland for these kinds of cases. We had no option but to find the required money to fight for Keri to fund this case. We were also told that even with supportive reports, the case could be lost in Court, which would result in loss. Not only the cost of the various reports commissioned but legal fees incurred by the hospital in defending the case would fall to us to be paid. That would result in us losing our family home. By taking on the hospital, we stood to lose everything.

We had no choice. Keri deserved justice to be done, and if that meant taking on another battle in the jungle of the HSE, so be it. This was one of many such battles in the years ahead. A big and risky battle but an exceptionally important one. We dug deep, and we wrote a cheque for €3,000 for the first of many expert Medico Legal reports. Our savings got whittled away by legal costs. Our lawyers got to work.

A few short days after our dismissal home from the hospital, I returned to our GP clinic. I was delirious with exhaustion and in utter despair. I explained to Dr Lawlor that I felt every door was being shut in our faces. I recounted the conversation with the doctor and was told I was spoiling my baby. I felt so useless and hopeless that I couldn't take the pain from Keri. My heart was absolutely broken. Days were dragging into nights, back to days again, without relief. There was little or no downtime, and I was lost as to what to do. Keri needed more help than I could give her. She was still in so much distress, and I felt nobody was listening. Dr Lawlor listened. She saw our distress. She picked up the telephone and made an appointment for us to consult with a Paediatrician in Clonmel for a second opinion. Our care was transferred to Clonmel Hospital, given its close proximity to our home in Fethard and, in particular, the fact that the God-sent Dr Eddie McGrath was based there.

We first met Dr Eddie McGrath on the 18th of March 2004, a day which transpired to be monumental in Keri's and all our lives. At long last, five months after her birth, not only were we placed in the care of an expert in respect of Keri's needs, but Dr McGrath was a man of such tenderness, compassion and intelligence. He listened attentively to everything I had to report on Keri's condition. Keri was, as usual, extremely distressed during this consultation. Dr McGrath could see that. I felt a weight lifting off my shoulders. We were no longer alone in our torment. Dr McGrath checked everything out. He concluded that, with the exception of *losec* (which was my idea), all medication Keri had been on over the previous five months was unsuitable. He immediately increased her *losec* and commenced her on *buscopan* to help her break wind. We were sent home to see if these changes made any difference, in the absence of which Dr McGrath would admit her for further investigations. The relentless misery remained despite these changes, but at least now I knew we had a plan and a medical professional who understood us.

Six days after our consultation with Dr McGrath, Keri was doing very badly, so I took her to Clonmel Hospital, where she screamed her little heart out. The staff at the front desk of the children's ward appeared quite taken aback by the condition Keri was in. Dr McGrath was called and arrived in a matter of minutes. Various tests were carried out, blood was taken, and we were escorted to a private room to settle Keri down for another hospital stay. An NG tube was fitted. This is a feeding tube which leads from the nose down to the stomach. She was five months old at this stage but still in newborn baby clothing. She didn't stand a chance if she couldn't be nourished, but we simply could not feed her.

Behind the door of that little room, the game face washed off with tears. I sobbed with exhaustion and bewilderment. I realized that I was feeling relieved to be in the hospital with my baby. I just didn't know how I could continue. I was at an all-time low point. Dr McGrath found me in that state, with Keri in my arms, in that familiar cycle of screaming, shaking and turning purple. He took Keri into his arms and spoke gently to her. He told her that he would do all he could to help her. He said, 'Your poor mother is exhausted. You have her wrecked'. I utterly broke down. The tears kept flowing. Every time I thought I was finished crying, more tears would flow.

I eventually pulled myself together. Now I had a medic that got it. Onwards and upwards. Large coffee in hand. Game face back on.

4

Pathways

That first night in Clonmel Hospital under the care of Dr McGrath can only be described as a nightmare. Keri was in such a bad way. Although it didn't feel like it at the time, it was also the start of a new and better chapter in Keri's life.

Nights for Keri, at this time, were the worst of her life. Her condition and distress came as a shock to the staff, but it had become our normality. In dire pain, she pulled her little legs up to her stomach and screamed until her face turned a reddish purple. She would then hold her breath in silence and scream again. It never stopped. I paced the floors of the ward with Keri in my arms, holding her close to me throughout the night, doing anything I could to settle her, just as I did during those long nights at home.

The following morning, Dr McGrath and his team came to see us on their ward rounds. In plain language, he explained to his team that Keri had Spastic Quadriplegic Cerebral Palsy arising from brain damage at her birth. None of these people had ever worked with a child with Keri's level of need, and some had never before seen a child with Cerebral Palsy. Dr McGrath impressed upon them that while these young doctors had worked for many years to gain their medical qualifications, it was essential that they listen to the parents, as they know the child best, being with them 24 hours every day. I explained how upsetting and frustrating it had been to be dismissed by so many professionals since Keri was born and how it was clear that none of this was in my imagination. I happily agreed with Dr McGrath to speak to these doctors later if they were to re-visit us. It was a good learning opportunity for them. Many did return later in the day. It was so refreshing and supportive to be given the space to openly and fully discuss Keri's difficulties.

Dr McGrath explored every avenue to get Keri the help she needed. During this hospital stay, he arranged for us to visit the Central Remedial Clinic (CRC) in Waterford to meet with their multi-disciplinary team. This included a speech/language therapist, an occupational physiotherapist and a dietician. We took Keri out of the hospital for the day to our first appointment in CRC, and we met the team. As she had been so sick, Keri was fed by NG tube at this time, but examination at the CRC revealed exactly why she wasn't able to feed. Keri was found to have an uncoordinated suck/swallow/breathe pattern, resulting in poor intake and extreme exhaustion. Given how important positioning is for eating, her whole-body extension pattern further significantly impaired her feeding (Keri would stretch out her entire body like a rigid wooden board). The biggest concern was that she would be unsafe when feeding, given the risk of aspiration (inhaling milk to her lungs, causing life-threatening pneumonia). A *Haberman* bottle, a special bottle for babies with impaired sucking ability, was ordered for Keri to be tried out. When we returned to the hospital, we updated Dr McGrath on what we had learned at CRC, a brilliant facility we were to return to for many years to come. We were so grateful to Dr McGrath for setting this up.

Keri remained in Clonmel Hospital for some time, and she was extremely unwell. Chalkie was working full time, and I stayed with Keri by day and by night. If she was somewhat settled, Chalkie would sit with her while I returned home for a quick shower. It was a really challenging time. Keri still cried so much, and the seizures were relentless. Everything was attempted in the search for relief for Keri. The nursing team were fantastic, and they did all they could for both of us. While our world was falling apart, these people carried us with their huge hearts. It meant so much to be given such time, kindness and much-needed reassurance that we were all doing everything we could for our little angel.

During this admission, a little girl from Fethard was admitted to the ward for a few nights. On one of those long and relentless nights, when the little girl was asleep, her mother, Fiona Dorney, popped her head around the door and said hello. I knew Fiona to see from Fethard. She sat with Keri and I and supported us both until 3am that night. Every night after that, once her little one was settled, Fiona would sit with us and keep us company. I barely knew Fiona, and she had no obligation whatsoever, but she showed such compassion to us at this time, and I will absolutely never forget it. The days and nights at Clonmel hospital continued to roll into one another. There were times when I wondered if we were ever going to return home. Keri remained very distressed.

Eventually, the much-anticipated *Haberman bottle* arrived at Clonmel hospital. While Keri was now nourished with NG feeding, it was so exciting to try normal feeding once again with a potentially appropriate bottle. The design of the *Haberman* allows tongue and gum pressure to release the milk, rather than by sucking (which Keri couldn't do). It also contains a valve to slowly release the feed, which prevents the child from becoming overwhelmed with milk and air (a massive problem for Keri). The bottle worked well for Keri. It was such a relief, after a long six months, to have a system to safely feed her. With the feeding situation improving, focus could now be turned to Keri's medication. This was important as Keri continued to suffer relentless seizures so violently that I was terrified her little heart would give up. However, as time went on, I learned of the extent of the force within her. A running family joke emerged that Keri was as stubborn as her mother! I became so grateful for the little fighter in her. Her little lion heart saved her, and it sustained her through these barbaric, relentless seizures.

Dr McGrath visited us for a chat. He enquired if I really understood Keri's condition. While I did have a fair idea, there was so much I didn't know. I asked him to be honest with me and to tell me everything. We all needed the full picture. Dr McGrath explained that Keri had very severe Spastic Quadriplegic Cerebral Palsy, which arose from brain damage. It was affecting all four limbs. He explained why she was suffering so much pain and stiffness in her little body. I recalled how Keri would often stiffen up like a plank of wood, and there would be no possible way to bend her. The whole-body extension pattern was causing so many difficulties. Dr McGrath enquired about the circumstances surrounding Keri's birth. I told him everything. He was astonished to hear about what we had gone through and categorically stated that her survival was an absolute miracle. Dr McGrath went on to tell me that Keri would have severe challenges for her entire life and that she may need a PEG tube inserted at some stage to feed her-a PEG is a flexible feeding tube which is surgically inserted into the stomach, though this would be far into the future. He encouraged us to try and feed her orally for as long as possible. I asked if Keri's condition would affect her life expectancy. To my horror, he said that it would. Dr McGrath explained that with the severity of her brain damage, she may not be expected to live longer than 18 years or possibly into her early 20s.

Nobody ever believes they will outlive their children, it isn't what nature intended, and it is not right. I felt sick to the pit of my stomach. Chalkie was devastated when I recounted the conversation with him later that evening.

As hard as it was to hear, I needed to know the truth of what we were living with and what the future held. I was so grateful to Dr McGrath for being so honest that day. There was a lot I did not know, but I needed to know about the life we had ahead of us.

I have the fondest memories of Dr McGrath. Every time he entered our room, before uttering a word, he would take Keri into his arms and gently speak to her. He was perfect for his profession; he was passionate about helping children, and he obviously loved his work. During one visit, Dr McGrath suggested that I consider writing a book about Keri. He felt the HSE should be made accountable for the mistakes made and expressed anger that this mistreatment happens all too often. He also felt huge frustration that parents like me are not listened to. I told him I was so often dismissed and made feel like I was the problem that I sometimes felt as if I was losing my mind. Dr McGrath wanted children like Keri to have a voice and be spoken for.

He couldn't stand the silence when so much was wrong with the system. I promised him I would write a book some day which I am now so proud of so thank you.

Dr McGrath showed us such support during our time in hospital, and he taught me about the proper standard of medical care I should expect and demand for myself and my family care, which, Dr McGrath said, should have been afforded to us from the very beginning. This was a vital education that armed me to carry Keri through many further battles in the years ahead.

During our time in Clonmel hospital, I was connected by another mother with a therapist by the name of Jimmy Conroy in Mountrath, County Laois. Jimmy is a faith healer, and I was told he settled distressed babies, particularly those with brain damage, and that while it would cause discomfort at first, it would give great relief in the long run. I made an appointment to bring Keri to see Jimmy, and we were lucky enough to be excused from the hospital for the day to attend. Chalkie drove us; I sat in the back with Keri, keeping a close, worried eye on her NG tube, which was drip-feeding her formula from a pre-prepared pouch. As we travelled down the long, narrow boreen grass growing up the central verge, we met another car coming against us, for whom we had to reverse. I reflected that this was the way we would now travel in life; two steps forward, one step back. I was very nervous about this meeting, as I had no idea what to expect. As we arrived at the end of the lane and pulled into his large tarmacadam driveway, I saw why he had been so highly recommended. There were cars on every corner, different families on their own unique journeys, all waiting to see Jimmy and get some relief. People were desperate to see him. We were told that the wait, no matter how long, would be worth it. We quickly learned that an organic queuing system arises in that countryside carpark, where those earliest get seen quickest, and one dare not attempt to skip ahead, no matter your allotted appointment time! While we waited, Chalkie and I heard phenomenal stories of what Jimmy had done for other children. We heard of a plain and ordinary man gifted with his work, full of knowledge and with a massive heart.

Our time came to introduce Keri to Jimmy. Despite how petrified I felt, we met an ordinary, kind-hearted, compassionate man who quickly put us all at ease. Jimmy's hands reminded me of Daddy's hands-there was a strength and gentleness to them. He carried no 'airs and graces'. We were welcomed to a small, simple treatment room with two chairs and a treatment plinth. Keri sat on my lap for the entirety of the session. As soon as Jimmy put his hands on Keri's head, he told us which side of her brain was damaged and why her body couldn't function like other babies. He explained that the body changes every seven years, and if he was to continue to treat Keri while making no promises, he may be able to help her symptoms. While we knew there was no miracle cure available, this gave us some badly needed hope for Keri. He treated Keri with a very firm massage, known as the 'rub down', with his thumb, 'thumb of steel', on her feet, hands, arms, stomach, back, neck and head. Jimmy explained that areas of distress, where a 'knot' arose, were being worked out by his thumbs to get things flowing again. While Keri screamed her little heart out throughout this first session, I told myself that it would be worth it. I was right.

This first session evolved into a beautiful lifelong relationship between Jimmy and Keri. The positive results after a session differed every time. Keri suffered badly from constipation, but there was always a bowel movement after a session with Jimmy, as indeed she enjoyed a reasonable night's sleep. Jimmy saw our good, our bad, our happy, our sad, our teary, our frustrated and our overjoyed days. In one particular session, Keri vomited all over the room during a treatment. Jimmy made no fuss about this. He simply wiped it up and continued to treat her. Keri adored him. No matter how many obstacles we had to overcome, Keri was treated by Jimmy every fortnight for the rest of her life.

The time came for Keri to be discharged home from Clonmel hospital - by then, it had been four weeks. Dr McGrath and the staff went through all the medication with us and connected us with as much support for Keri as they possibly could. Dr McGrath generously shared his mobile number and organised a review in a week's time. Our discharge home was exciting and terrifying in equal measure.

When Chalkie brought us home, I was so grateful for the spotlessly clean, warm home which awaited us. Once Keri was settled, I visited our local Pharmacist, Jimmy O Sullivan, with Keri's prescription. Jimmy and his wonderful team provided an incredible service to Keri throughout her lifetime. She was a complex case and so sensitive to medication, so there was a lot of figuring out to do, but Jimmy never gave up. The over and above service to deliver medication to us if we couldn't leave the house further speaks of his generosity and professionalism. Keri loved visiting the pharmacy as she was always treated like absolute royalty and always admired and spoken to so kindly. Keri loved the attention and lapped it all up.

As we settled in at home, I received a call from Maura Lonergan in the HSE, who said she was sent all of Keri's details from Dr McGrath and that she would like to visit us. From that day on, Maura became a huge part of our lives. She frequently visited us and was so generous with her time and experience. She organised funding for 'home help' hours from the HSE for Keri and constantly checked in to see if there was any more that could be done for us.

She offered support, advice and information, which was so helpful and reassuring. She never rushed off, giving us as much time as we needed-especially if Keri was having a day of relentless crying. Maura has a heart as big as a mountain. I really could have done with her in our lives from day one.

One of the supports organised by the HSE was the Early Intervention Team, which brought Mary Nolan Maher into our lives. From Keri's 7th month, Mary called on a weekly basis and engaged with Keri in a playful way to encourage her to interact. Keri warmed to Mary, who always made sure the sessions were enjoyable, even on a bad day when Keri didn't seem impressed! Mary also had many superb tips for me as to how to make life easier for us all.

Throughout these early years, we continued to stay in very close contact with Dr McGrath, Dr Lawlor GP, Dr Condon GP and the team at CRC. Keri also saw Valerie Cantwell, Physiotherapist, on a weekly basis. We depended on all of these people so much to do the best we could for Keri, as she required help in every aspect of her little body and her life.

At the CRC, we attended some really helpful feeding clinics, where Mairead, Damhnait and Cliona regularly investigated Keri's intake, output and growth measurements, offering very helpful advice on how to safely feed Keri while helping her develop oral-motor skills. They taught us how to spoon feed Keri, and they monitored her closely as time went on. It was an incredible service. In time, we became adept at feeding Keri successfully so that she could gain weight and enjoy the satisfaction of a good meal. She began to gain weight.

In June 2004, when Keri was 8 months old, we attended Dr Bourke, Consultant Gastroenterologist in Crumlin. Treatment of Keri's stomach issues was tricky. While the vomiting had subsided by then, the screaming continued. Dr Bourke wasn't convinced that Keri was suffering from Gastroesophageal Reflux. He suspected her brain injury was affecting her stomach in some other way, so he sought the opinion of a Paediatric Neurologist. Keri's was a difficult case. Ultimately, it was felt that Keri was suffering a neurological reaction to the food hitting the *villi*-the little hair like fibres on the inside of the gut-which was causing her distress. To my mind, that was a gut-brain link associated with her brain injury. I found that by strictly following the Kinesiology diet, by carefully and slowly feeding Keri non-acidic food and drink (but never together-drinks, were always taken separately to meals), we kept the reflux symptoms at bay as much as possible.

This was an incredibly busy time. There were so many appointments for Keri-GP, Consultant, Hospital, CRC, Osteopath, Jimmy Conroy, and Play Therapist. However, the intervention and help was working. What started at 20 hours of crying per day, frequently up to 23 hours, had reduced to 10 hours. For us, and especially for Keri, that was an incredibly easier life than what we endured in those first 6 months.

After approximately 9 months, a further blessing came upon us in the form of Dr Condon, GP, who took over Keri's care in our local GP clinic as Dr Lawlor was only covering maternity leave. From then on, Dr Condon remained Keri's GP for the rest of her life. She jumped on our rollercoaster with enthusiasm and interest in Keri. With the help of Dr Fuller, Judy (Nurse) and the girls at the desk, Keri was treated as a princess; always prioritised, always protected. Keri tugged on their heartstrings - she had that effect on people; she brought out the very best in them, and in turn, they brought out the best in her.

5

Roly Poly

Money was becoming a huge worry. I had no income. In view of Keri's condition, there was no way I could return to work. As I had been self-employed (at the sandwich bar), I was not entitled to a maternity benefit payment. The mortgage and bills piled up, and this added to our worries. While Keri was an inpatient in Clonmel hospital, I was advised that I was entitled to a Domiciliary Care Allowance and a Carers Allowance from the Department of Social Welfare. While these payments eased the pressure somewhat, we remained flat broke. On one particular day, I didn't have the price of a coffee in my purse. A lot of Keri's treatments were private - not only were the fees expensive, but the travel costs quickly mounted up, too. I didn't tell my family about this financial strain, and I was too embarrassed.

Out of the blue, my prayers were answered. Caitriona Davey, a friend of mine from my time working at Dawn Fresh Foods, contacted me to ask if I would be interested in childminding for her. At the time, Caitriona had two girls, Kate and Carrie, who were 4 and 2. Frankly, I didn't know how I would manage everything, but I agreed to give it a go. My biggest fear was that Kate and Carrie wouldn't react well to Keri, as she was still screaming so much, but we all quickly got used to each other. What really helped in this settle-in stage was how easy-going their mother, Caitriona, was; she appreciated what I was doing to support her family. There was a lot of organising and early mornings to make it work. For my own peace of mind, I had to have the children's dinner prepared before they arrived at 7:15am if possible because I never knew what kind of day Keri would have. If Keri was in pain, I would have to devote my attention to her almost exclusively. As long as the children had full bellies, I could relax in the knowledge that they would be content and satisfied. There were constant appointments for Keri, but the girls didn't mind coming along. They were easy-going children, like their lovely Mum and Dad.

The new childminding arrangements immediately made a huge financial difference-I was now able to take Keri for all the private treatments she needed, and I never felt under the same pressure to make ends meet. Furthermore, it allowed us to splash out on occasional Sundays and have dinner out, which was fantastic. Another massive bonus was the friendship that grew between Caitriona and I; she has always been a huge support to me, and to this day, I really value our friendship.

Carrie and Kate became best buddies with Keri but also little therapists for her. There were certain exercises that had to be done with Keri twice daily, every day, in order to stretch out her muscles and encourage her development. While I would do these activities on my own with Keri in the morning, the afternoon sessions with the Davey children were far more fun for Keri, which, in turn, made things far easier for me. Kate and Carrie loved therapy time with Keri. One of the tasks was to lie Keri on her back and encourage her to roll onto her tummy. The girls would egg Keri on, singing.

Roly poly, roly poly, roll, roll, roll.
Roly poly, roly poly, roll, roll, roll.
Roly poly, roly poly, roll, roll, roll.
Roly poly, roly poly, roll, roll, roll.

All the while, the girls would be on a mat on the floor with her, rolling around, demonstrating how to do it, shrieking with excitement, and encouraging Keri to follow suit. When Keri would eventually roll over, the girls would clap and shout *hooray*! My heart would burst with joy and gratitude in witnessing such love, praise and friendship for my baby from such tiny children rolling around together on the floor.

Keri needed a lot of equipment, which changed and grew with her as time went on. Three of her most important pieces of kit were her specialised buggy, her stander and her specialised high chair for feeding and activities.

Joanne McHugh in the HSE Occupational Therapy Department provided all the equipment she needed in ongoing consultation with the Central Remedial Clinic, who reviewed Keri's needs and provided various recommendations. Keri absolutely hated her stander. In these early years, aged 2 to 7, she used a Leckey prone stander, which she would lean against.

In simple terms, a Stander is a standing frame on wheels (with brakes) that a person with quadriplegia cerebral palsy is strapped to at the feet, knees, thighs and abdomen/chest in an upright position. In the case of the Leckey prone stander, the child is settled onto it, table in front, strapped in from behind, with the support of leg splints. It could be described as an all-body splint to affect a standing position. Standers are designed to encourage muscle and bone development, promote the use of the legs and lift a person from the wheelchair level to encourage social interaction. Keri found being in the stander extremely difficult, and she absolutely hated it. Getting her into it was very tricky as she would push against me and make it as awkward as she could manage, the determined little monkey! I had to be cruel to be kind; there was no choice.

Once in the stander, Kate, Carrie, and I would prance around like lunatics, ringing bells, singing and dancing, doing anything at all just to keep her distracted. We would wrap bells around Keri's hands and shake them, all the while singing songs. Over time, we managed to extend the length of time that Keri would tolerate her stander to 20 minutes or an exceptional 30 minutes on a really good day. This progress was down, in no small way, to the help of the little Davey therapists!

Another activity to encourage Keri to lift her head whilst lying on her tummy (in prone) was to lay her face down on her Peanut Roll (a large, inflatable rubber physio roll in the shape of a monkey nut). Keri would lie in the middle of it, and I would roll her back and forth until her feet would hit the floor to gently encourage putting weight on her legs. Lying over the peanut roll helped Keri develop her neck and back muscles, all vitally important to assist with maintaining a proper feeding position. The peanut roll was also a huge source of fun for Kate and Carrie, who loved nothing more than to scoot around on it.

Keri's mode of transport was, in the early days, a 7-seater car to allow for the large special-needs buggy and adequate seating for the other children. Later, from the age of 5, when Keri got her first wheelchair, we upgraded to a bus, whereby we would seat her in her special seat, placing her wheelchair into the boot. Later, when we upgraded her wheelchair to a larger size, we purchased a transit van with windows and wheelchair accessibility. This bus allowed us to roll Keri into the vehicle without taking her out of her wheelchair, securely fastening her to the anchor points and allowing her to see out and travel safely and comfortably.

The Davey children didn't see Keri as different, and they loved her exactly as she was. They became our family, and we became theirs. When Keri would succeed in a task at physio, their loud and loving commotion brought out Keri's greatest, widest beaming smiles. She did her best for them. They got the best out of her. They learned empathy and compassion, all the while having great fun. Everyone's lives were enriched.

I have such incredible memories of our trips on Keri's bus. As soon as we got on the bus, all the children would ask whose turn it was to sit beside Keri. They all loved her bones of her. Everyone loved music, so the tunes were always on. We bopped along to CD's like Dirty Dancing, Mika and the NOW albums. It became a huge sing-song, a bus full of lunatics, and it was brilliant fun.

Teeth were an ongoing source of brutality for poor Keri over many years. As each new milk tooth cut through her little gums, an infection would flare up, causing her huge pain and discomfort. For every tooth that appeared, Keri had an admission to the hospital for treatment. The screaming was relentless during these times.

When Keri was up to it, Chalkie took her walking, and she absolutely loved it. She loved hearing the birds chirping, the cows mooing and having the free air blow in her little face. Her little curly haired head was so cute, bopping along in the buggy; she was just so perfect.

When Keri was seven months old, we had a surprise visit to our door. Jonathan and Marie-Ann Irwin, founders and directors of the Jack and Jill Foundation, introduced themselves. They explained that they had learned of Keri while attending a local event in Fethard and decided to visit to offer help. We heard all about what the Foundation was for and how it came about. We learned about their beloved little boy Jack, who had tragically passed away, and how they honoured his inspiring life by setting up a Foundation to help other families. Following the visit, Jonathan and Marie-Ann connected us with their area nursing manager, Mary Jo, who allocated nursing hours to us, available after we found ourselves the right person to care for Keri. Eventually, my very good friend Marita introduced me to a very special lady by the name of Cora, who had experience in the Noonan Centre, now known as Scoil Aonghusa, a local school for children with special needs.

When Cora and I met, we clicked immediately. All I wanted was a kind-hearted, gentle person who was willing to devote themselves to Keri while in her presence. We agreed to give it a go. I trained Cora in every aspect of Keri's needs, and Cora worked really hard to learn how best to care for Keri. Most importantly, Keri and Cora bonded immediately. Feeding was a tricky point, as we knew it would be; it had taken us so many months to get it right. Cora persisted and eventually mastered it, too. Once she was competent and confident in feeding Keri, my life changed for the better. After the initial few months of training, I was able to leave home with peace of mind knowing she was safe with a suitably trained kind hearted carer.

Cora was like an angel sent from heaven. She allowed me a few hours a week to leave the house in confidence, stretch my legs, recharge myself and restock the fridge and cupboards of our kitchen. The Jack and Jill Foundation changed our lives for the better.

In May 2005, when Keri was 18 months old, she was admitted to the hospital for an overnight EEG (electroencephalogram). This test records brain activity and abnormalities of brainwave patterns. It was felt at this stage that Keri was not, in fact, suffering from epilepsy at all but rather was suffering from extreme muscle spasms, which appeared like epilepsy. Keri was gradually weaned off the epilepsy medication. (It was some years later that we learned Keri did, in fact, have epilepsy all along, but the *Buccal Midazolam* she was taking long term had masked the epilepsy, making them appear like spasms). Given the severity of her muscle spasms, Keri was referred to Dr Noelle Cassidy, Consultant Orthopaedic Surgeon, to discuss administering *Botox* to her muscles. When injected into the muscle in tiny amounts, it can stop or reduce muscle spasms by blocking nerve signals to the muscle, so the hope was that it would give Keri some relief. Unfortunately, arising from lengthy waiting lists, it wasn't until early the following year that we met with Dr Cassidy in relation to this. The HSE is blighted by long, slow, agonising waiting lists.

Later in the summer of 2005, we were lucky enough to be given the sponsored opportunity to bring Keri to Lourdes with the Cashel & Emily diocese. We didn't hesitate to go. Lourdes is a place known to heal, and I personally felt if it would give us some reassurance, some faith and direction in our path with Keri's condition, then it would be worthwhile. Moreover, I was hopeful it would bring relief to Keri's suffering. Lourdes was very peaceful; there was a spiritual energy there that was so special, and I felt a weight lifting off me during those days.

It was the most beautiful and breath-taking holiday, and we met some wonderful people, all on a path like ours, all at a down to earth level that often comes with great human suffering. We dined with other families and got to spend time together, exchanging stories, advice and wisdom. There was a sing-song session in the evenings in the reception area of the hotel, which brought so much joy to so many. Keri was so calm in Lourdes, her sleep was much better there, and she seemed so content for those few days. I felt as if she was just inhaling all the love and peace surrounding her, and it was doing her so much good. As soon as we arrived home, we started saving our money to go again the following year. It is said that if you visit Lourdes three years in a row, it is even more helpful for a patient. Ultimately, we managed to do that, visiting Lourdes with Keri in 2005, 2006 and in 2007 when Lucy arrived too. I genuinely believe these pilgrimages really did help Keri.

6

Smiles

Every second morning, I prepared meals, especially for Keri. She tolerated small portions of blended, smooth foods only; lumps would make her gag and vomit. Her dinners consisted of cod, lamb or chicken with carrots, broccoli and rice, cooked together with an organic gluten-free stock cube, blended in its own juices. For dessert, Keri would have an Alpro soya yoghurt, heated slightly (Keri couldn't tolerate any cold foods). Keri loved to eat Milupa Semolina and Honey, Milupa Crispies and Milupa Rice. Milupa products were a lifeline as they were, for a period, all she could eat and enjoy. They were easy to prepare, nutritious and useful for feeding when on the road to therapies.

We fed Keri in a special needs high chair, the Leckey II. It had a harness to keep her hips in place, cushioned-chest straps to keep her upright and a headrest to support her in a correct and safe position as she fed. Feeding was a slow process. Before starting, I would use a little vibrating device around her mouth so that she would know, with that sensation, that it was feeding time. Each spoonful had to be fully swallowed before another could be introduced to her little mouth. I used a Tommy Tippee spoon as it is very soft and small. I would put the spoon in her mouth with a little cluster of food and tip it down on her tongue very gently. That would prompt Keri to bring the food back to her mouth and swallow it when she was ready. I then gently massaged, with the longside of my index finger, from chin to throat, to remind her to move the food back her mouth and down her throat. Keri required quietness and patience during this time. If she was distracted during feeding, she wouldn't be able to concentrate on working the food back in her mouth with her tongue and safely swallowing it. She couldn't be rushed. Before the next mouthful, her mouth always had to be perfectly clear to avoid aspirating into her lungs. On a slow day, a meal could take up to 45 minutes. Drinking could not take place at the same time as feeding, as it would overwhelm her little system.

It took years and years of trial and error, with many tears and countless vomits, but we eventually got the right formula and feeding technique in place for Keri. Eventually, Keri absolutely adored her meals, and it was such a joy to feed her, especially after the initial brutality of her feeding as a small baby. She couldn't run around a park like other children, so a nice warm meal was one of her few pleasures in life. If I had a euro for every time it was suggested to me that I should just PEG feed Keri, I would have quickly become a very rich lady. It would, of course, have been easier to PEG feed her, and it would, of course, have been faster, but Keri loved her food, and it brought me so much joy to see this. It took time, patience, and perseverance to get meals into her, little spoon by little spoon, but she enjoyed it, and I enjoyed the intimacy and pleasure of feeding her. That said, there is no judgment for any other feeding situation-ultimately Keri had to be PEG-fed too, when oral feeding became unsafe some years later, but while I could feed Keri safely and successfully (some would say, painfully slowly), this was exactly what I was going to do. It was Keri that mattered, not me. I could guzzle a sandwich down in two minutes if I needed to. Any joy we could bring her simply had to come first.

In the summer of 2005, overflowing with gratitude for the help Cora was giving me, we decided to do something to give back to the Jack and Jill Foundation, which was funding this assistance. After some consideration, it was decided to host a Valentine's Ball at the Hotel Minella in Clonmel the following February 2006. I approached John Nallen, the owner of Hotel Minella. He overwhelmed me with his generosity. Having years of experience in organising events, he shared so much valuable advice as to what I needed to do.

A date was set, and we organised a Garda permit to sell tickets to prove it was a genuine charitable event. Every door approached was easily opened; the local people of Fethard were so decent and kind with support and offered to help. When I approached businesses looking for support or donations, I never brought Keri with me, as I would have considered that disrespectful to both Keri and the business owner. Cora or Chalkie minded Keri for me during this time. Chalkie called in his contacts, too. Wherever our friends went, they sought and received donations for the raffle. For first prize, we were facilitated by Susan at the 'Town & County' shop in Fethard to arrange at cost price the delivery of a replica rocking horse that the late Queen Elizabeth enjoyed as a little girl. It was a beautiful piece.

The event was a resounding success. I relaxed and enjoyed it, reassured that Cora was looking after Keri perfectly well at home. Cora would call me if there was any problem. People were so generous, and it was genuinely great fun. The highlight for me was undoubtedly the honour of having Dr Eddie McGrath and his wife attend. Every wonderful prize in the raffle, gorgeous Peter Curling paintings, vouchers and hampers were all donated as gifts to the event. A wonderful couple, Kevin and Donna Buckley, won the rocking horse. They are blessed with two beautiful, healthy children of their own who would have been delighted to receive the prize, but the Buckleys insisted that Keri have it. I was so grateful for their generosity, and Keri adored that rocking horse. Gestures like this meant the world to us. They helped us through the tough times to remember the love and support out there for us. The Jack and Jill Foundation were delighted with the funds raised (€56,000), and I received a gorgeous follow up note of thanks from Jonathan.

I knew first hand that those funds would be put to great use. The home care support was such an incredible help, but there were other offerings from Jack and Jill, most notably, the very special annual summer events. During these mini-festivals, service users, their families and friends are welcomed with open arms to a large venue where children, no matter their disability, would enjoy music, face painting, balloons, massage, ice-cream, food, drinks, and entertainment. Facilities were meticulously put in place to ensure all the various additional needs were met. Jonathan Irwin and the nurses would also attend. These were wonderful days where all the families got to connect with others in similar situations, and the primary aim of the day was to see as many smiles as possible. Keri managed to make it to three of these events over her lifetime. Unfortunately, her health didn't allow her to go annually, but she adored these days out, and it was so uplifting to see so many happy faces on children faced with so many daily struggles.

Since the prior summer, we had been looking forward to our meeting with Dr Noelle Cassidy in the Central Remedial Clinic in Clontarf to discuss Botox for Keri's muscle spasms. By January 2006, when the meeting took place, the spasms had become much more severe and distressing for Keri. We discussed everything. Dr Cassidy expertly considered all options to alleviate Keri's pain. Dr

Cassidy wasn't convinced Botox would help. I eventually persuaded her, promising her that if it didn't work, at least we would have tried, and I would leave her alone at that point! She agreed to give it a go. Soon after, Keri received her first set of Botox injections, and to our surprise, they were very successful, so these were repeated every 12 weeks in Temple Street Hospital. Dr Cassidy was amazing, excellent at her job and very down to earth. On each occasion, Dr Cassidy would pinpoint different areas of Keri's body where she would receive the most benefit from the treatment. While initially Keri would require a general anaesthetic for the procedure, we soon learned that this caused immense distress and stomach upset for her. Luckily, as time went on, Keri became accustomed to the injections, such that they could be done with her awake. She was a tough cookie! Later, the injections were administered at the National Orthopaedic Hospital in Cappagh, Dublin, which was far easier to reach and a lot less stressful. Mammy always came with us for these visits to Cappagh for support. As we had to be in the hospital at 0745hrs, we usually stayed in a hotel the night before. The injections really helped Keri, and the spasms came under control. Our little fighter got some respite from her suffering.

Keri's busy schedule of Botox, Kinesiology, Cranial Osteopathy, Play Therapy, Jimmy Conroy, and Physiotherapy reaped the ultimate reward. Keri began to smile and enjoy herself. She began to respond far better to her

Physiotherapy and OT sessions, and she was making visible progress. Our little warrior had survived her grueling battle with muscle spasms, and she began to thrive. Close friends were now regularly visiting Keri for comfort, feeling better during a bad day to have spent some time with her, Keri being a person who makes the world a better place. Being in Keri's company became a therapy for those lucky enough to be closest to her. A new chapter had begun.

7

Preschooler

Those busy days and long nights translated into fast but tender years, submerged in love and awe of Keri's strength and resilience. 2006 brought us to Keri's third year when she was to begin pre-school. While I was relieved that she was offered a place in *Lus na Greine*, a wonderful early learning facility for children with additional needs, I was also anxious as to how she and I would cope with being apart from each other. However, I knew she was ready for school and that we both needed it. *Lus na Greine* had every service Keri required in the school setting. The staff were incredible. This step forward was for her highest good. My heart was in my mouth, bringing her in on the first day, but I had to think of what was best for Keri. This opened up a whole new world for all of us.

Over her time in *Lus na Greine,* a facility run by the Brothers of Charity, Keri could not have been in more capable hands. Manager Caitriona, Occupational Therapist Bridget, Nurses Marguerite, Caroline, Michelle and all the team were all incredibly devoted, patient, and compassionate. They were experienced professionals who worked hand in hand with the parents for every child's best interests. I fully engaged in a diary system with the school, where I would report on feeding, sleep and general form, and they would do likewise as to how Keri was on any given day. Every piece of equipment that Keri required at home was also available as a 'double set' for her use at school. This was hugely reassuring.

The early months were really tough on everyone. Initially, I spent a lot of time with the team, showing exactly how Keri was to be fed and watered. While at the outset, I was allowed to stay for short periods, I did eventually have to leave so that everyone could get to know each other. This was really difficult, especially when Keri was still crying and distressed as I left the room on some occasions. Keri was confronted with ill health at this time; she was in a lot of pain. Oftentimes, I would be called back to collect her early, such was her persistent screaming. The team kept her in school as long as they could, but as it got towards lunchtime, the feeling was (rightly) that Keri was too upset to be fed, so I would take her home and get her settled before lunch on those days.

Given the enormity of her health challenges, settling Keri into school took two entire years. Every time a tooth would break through her gums, Keri would develop an infection, requiring admission to hospital on IV medication. It would take weeks to re-settle her, only for another tooth to erupt. It was so cruel to witness this additional and relentless burden for Keri.

It wasn't until Keri was heading towards 5 years old, that she was able to really enjoy all that pre-school had to offer. For this reason, a decision was so kindly made to allow Keri a further year in *Lus na Greine* to really benefit from it. This was the right decision for Keri. She blossomed hugely in that last year. By then, she was able to enjoy the full service of play therapy, music, singing time, stories, Physiotherapy, sensory activities and fun with her switch toys. She went to and from school on the bus, driven by Christy or Liam, treated like royalty on board with her special little friend Tamara. She also developed a really extraordinary friendship with James, her 'boyfriend' over all the years, whose mother Linda became one of my best friends. When Keri and James were together, each of their eyes would light up. They had a really unique connection.

After school, Keri would come home and immediately have a drink (as she couldn't eat and drink simultaneously, this was very important at this time). We would then have a long cuddle on the comfy chair together, Keri on my lap, cuddled into my chest. This spot, in this position, was our happy place, where we were both blissfully happy and at home.

At this time, Keri's teeth were regularly reviewed by the paediatric dental team at the HSE clinic in Clonmel. Keri was on a particular medication, *Vallergan,* which was causing tooth decay. It was advised that her 8 baby molars were to be removed to allow for her adult molars to come through easily, avoiding compaction or further pain. We went with the advice. Keri was referred to Dublin for the surgery, and thankfully, she recovered well from these extractions.

I continued to look after Kate and Carrie. If I had to collect Keri early from the school, I would load them into the seven seater to collect Keri. I was so lucky that the Davey kids were so easy-going that I could do this if I needed to. In the afternoons, everyone would either travel with us for Keri's various private therapy appointments or get involved at home with her Physiotherapy and occupational therapy exercises. It was a team effort, and everyone played a really important and special part. It was with great joy we learned in 2005 that Kate and Carrie were to become big sisters to twins! Caitriona gave birth to Emily and Jack in March 2006, and they soon also came under my care.

In September 2006, Noelle gave birth to a magnificent little girl, Kaycie, and I was honoured to be asked to be her Godmother, a role I have ever since cherished and treasured. Our colourful, playful, united tribe was growing in strength and numbers!

Dr McGrath rang me in late 2006. Keri was three years old by then, and there wasn't a day I didn't think of Dr McGrath and all he had done for us. He had the saddest of news. While he had taken leave to focus on his health some time back, his battle with cancer had been relentless, and he was losing the fight. True to form, he asked all about Keri and reminded me of my promise to write this book.

Dr McGrath passed away on the 28th of December, 2006. Even in his passing, he helped us understand Keri. Keri was as good as gold in the church, and it was like she knew how special a man he was. After the funeral, Keri was due to take a bottle but refused point blank. I took her out of the bus and wheeled her around a clothes shop named Sasha at the time that we were parked outside. I noticed Keri had been looking at a particular dress in the window. I found two lovely dresses for Keri and could see that she liked them. I told her I would make a deal with her; that if she drank her bottle for me, I would get her one of the dresses. I took her to the back of the shop where it was quiet, well, she necked her bottle in record time! I was thrilled. We had struck our first bargain. I couldn't have been happier. I picked up both dresses, and I asked her to show me which one she would prefer. Her eyes veered to one but looked back occasionally to the second, and this happened on a couple of occasions. I was so thrilled with her showing me her preferences and ability to engage in a bribe that I bought them both for her! I knew at that moment that our Keri had plenty of personality, clear preferences, and an ability to strike a deal in order to get her way. She had me wrapped completely around her little finger. It was a massive milestone.

Dr McGrath had taken his rightful place in heaven. He will never be forgotten as one of the most inspirational people I have ever met. He left behind an enormous legacy; he saved my beautiful Keri, and he showed us the way we should expect to be treated. I pray that he has been reunited with Keri in heaven, and I often think of the two of them together in heaven, spurring me on to complete this book and that I thank you both from the bottom of my heart. I can only hope I have done you both very proud.

8

Sisterhood

The medico-legal investigation by the solicitors continued. The records were taken up from the hospital, collated, photocopied and couriered to England for the preparation of an expert medial report. Our first report was completed by an eminent Consultant Obstetrician and Gynaecologist in England who examined all of Keri's notes in detail. He also considered my own recollection of events.

The report concluded in the strongest of terms that there was obvious negligence in the care afforded to Keri during my labour and her delivery. He identified massive systems failures, which left signs of fetal compromise to go unnoticed. Most notably, a failure to properly monitor and record my uterine contractions with Keri's heart rate on the CTG monitor was reported upon. Had this vitally important data been understood, Keri's severe distress would have been identified, and the appropriate steps taken to arrange an urgent caesarean section far earlier, saving her from catastrophic and irreversible brain damage.

In other words, Keri was in distress during the labour. The staff did not act upon it. This failure caused Keri to be delivered almost dead, with a cord wrapped around her neck.

Having read the report, I was tormented at the thought of the cord hurting Keri, that this thing was pulling at her while she was inside me, strangling her and hurting her. Even now, I still feel guilty that this was happening to Keri, and I couldn't do anything to protect her from it.

With negligence now established with this first report, it was time to investigate causation. What that involved was asking a Paediatric Neurologist to examine Keri, consider the contents of the obstetric report and establish if the negligence during the course of her delivery had *caused* her brain damage. Cerebral Palsy arises for multiple reasons, but the purpose of this report was to rule out any other cause, be it Infection, Genetics, Prematurity or other reasons. We dug deep to find a further €3,000 to fund this second report, paid it to the solicitors and got back to work at home. We couldn't afford this report, nor indeed the last one, but we didn't have a choice in the matter. We had to get to the truth of what happened, Keri, and why it happened.

In the summer of 2006, when Keri was almost three years old, I learned about Kinesiology and how it may be very beneficial for children in Keri's predicament. I was connected to a therapist. I spoke with Valerie, who organised his appointments for the first time by telephone, recounting the events leading to Keri's brain injury and the distress she had since suffered. As Keri was so small and in so much distress, it was decided that she would be treated through me in the first instance, in a process known as surrogacy.

I lay on the treatment bed, and the therapist put Keri's pyjamas (which she had worn the previous night) on top of my stomach and employed a technique to bring Keri into my body. It was described to me as surrogacy. Keri was at home with her father all this time. The therapist worked on Keri's body through mine. In so doing, he could feel what was happening to her, where her difficulties were. All the while, I felt Keri's energies inside me. I could feel her pain; her every muscle that ached her. As distressing as it was to know her level of physical pain, the insight was so helpful for compassion, for understanding her and what she was going through. I was crying, but they were Keri's tears. He asked where the tears came from, and I replied that Keri was crying because she could not run around with her friends. He went through the whole birth process with her (through me) as she understood exactly what happened to her. He did this to clear the hurt from her body. The technique he used was to say, 'I forget the upset I feel about not being able to run around with my friends' while doing the tapping technique. He kept asking what number sadness, and eventually, it came down from ten to zero. Then there was a massive deep breath, which I took involuntarily, after which I confirmed that Keri was fine now, that the sadness was gone. In that way, he cleared her of negative energies, thereby allowing her space to receive good energies to heal her.

I was gobsmacked. I had plainly felt Keri's pain, her every muscle. It was both amazing and distressing in equal measure. Feeling Keri's anguish in that moment, I connected with her on an even deeper level. During that time, Keri was at home with Chalkie, who later told me that while she was distressed initially, she soon relaxed and became very peaceful. I was sent home with a list of nutritional supplements to buy for Keri, together with a list of foods that she was intolerant to. I was also given a list of pressure points to work on at home with Keri directly in order to further help her.

Keri decided that she rather liked being inside me during these 'surrogacy' sessions. She loved the comfort of it. It was, for her, like being back in the womb. At the end of one particular session, the kinesiologist couldn't get her out of me. The extraction process took 45 minutes or so. I started to get anxious, but we got there. After that episode and for many further years, Keri attended Kinesiology treatments herself. There was no way we were trying surrogacy again, as we worried what the next time might bring trying to get Keri out of me. I stuck religiously to the directions given, I just knew from the surrogacy experience that this therapy would help her live a more comfortable and happy life. That absolutely proved to be the case.

When Keri was three years old, Chalkie and I discussed having another child. Before I would even consider things further, I needed to be certain that we would both be safe. I arranged an appointment with Dr Hack, a Consultant Obstetrician at Clonmel Hospital, at that time. I recalled what had happened during Keri's birth, how I wanted another child but not unless it was to be delivered safely by caesarean. Dr Hack was so understanding. He said that absolutely, under the circumstances, I could have a caesarean section, and he later arranged a visit to the theatre so that I would be familiar with the environment. Having been reassured, I was then lucky enough to fall pregnant very quickly. I was absolutely thrilled.

During my pregnancy with Lucy, I felt relaxed and happy. I showed Keri my bump and talked often with her about her new baby brother or sister. I was convinced it was a boy. I was so excited. The pregnancy was perfect. I felt healthy and blessed to be pregnant again.

It was during my pregnancy with Lucy that it became apparent that there was a lot of strain on our marriage. I was feeling immensely lonely, unsupported and unloved. Chalkie and I were leading completely separate lives. He was at work by day and in the garden in the evening. I spent my days and nights with Keri, keeping on top of the house and minding the children. We didn't eat meals together, and there was no affection. I tried my best to feel positive, and I dearly hoped it would all be OK. There was another baby on the way, we were both doing our best in the circumstances we were in, but the gap between us was widening further.

While I was pregnant with Lucy, Caitriona returned to work after maternity leave on the twins, so I now had the four gorgeous Davey children and my princess Keri under my care. It was a busy time in the house, and Keri still had not settled in school. There were many days I had to bundle all four of them into my car to collect Keri if she was having a bad day. This was just part and parcel of life.

A date was set at thirty-eight weeks for my elective caesarean section. Caitriona made alternative arrangements with her parents for three weeks of childminding cover while I took some maternity leave. Chalkie took a week off work to look after Keri while I was in hospital. I was convinced we were having a boy, so much so that I brought a little blue outfit into the hospital for the baby! My sister Fionnuala was only delighted to accompany me in the theatre for the delivery and support.

Lucy's birth, on the 20th of February 2007, was absolutely beautiful. I was given an epidural but was fully awake. I felt them tugging and manipulating my belly to get the baby out. While I imagined it may be scary, it was just perfect. I loved every minute of it. It showed me how magnificent a birth can be, and it was an incredibly healing experience for me.

After Lucy was delivered, there was a silence for a few seconds before she cried. That first cry was the best sound

I have ever heard. Lucy had swallowed meconium (a baby's first bowel motion ingested during delivery). While she was allowed back to the ward with me to meet her father, she was then taken to the Special Care Baby Unit to be monitored.

The time alone in the hospital room without either of my girls was torture. I felt I couldn't breathe without them. I couldn't eat or sleep, and I was highly emotional. Having Lucy in the Special Care Baby Unit brought back terrible memories of Keri's time in the neonatal unit, and although I knew Lucy was going to be perfectly fine, I felt completely overwhelmed.

The fantastic staff at Clonmel hospital provided me with a private room so that Keri could visit me. We arranged the week off school for Keri, and Chalkie brought her into me each day. Chalkie would very gently lift Keri onto my lap in the bed as I was quiet sore after the section, and we would have a snuggle, her face on my chest, our happy place, together-where we were at home and at ease, no matter where we were. Her departure each day was so painful. I imagine the hormones played their part, too; I was a blubbering mess saying our goodbyes. The staff saw how upset I was, so I persuaded the doctor to discharge me home a day early. They suggested I would do well to have the break in the hospital, but I just couldn't wait to get safely home and spend the days and nights with our two gorgeous girls.

Lucy's homecoming was fantastic for everyone, with the exception of three and a half year old Keri! She had her own very strong opinions on the matter, and she wasn't afraid to voice them! At that time, Keri was still sleeping in our bedroom when she did sleep, as I needed to be able to attend to her quickly when she had a spasm. The plan was for the four of us to co-sleep in the short term. As we placed Lucy's Moses basket in our bedroom, I showed Keri where her little sister Lucy would be sleeping. Immediately, Keri started shouting incessantly. We were shocked! Chalkie took the basket out of the room. Keri stopped shouting. Chalkie brought the basket back in, and the shouting resumed. We tried it a third time, and Keri had the exact same reaction. A clear cause and effect! We were delighted to see Keri express herself without words. Despite her brain injury, we could see for the first time how aware Keri was of her surroundings and preferences. It was wonderful. Needless to say, Keri got her way, and Lucy was put into her own bedroom from the first night. Chalkie and I took turns to sleep with each of the girls in the separate bedrooms. In some ways, Keri's reaction was reflective of our marital situation. We were separate by day, and now, we were separate by night.

Lucy was such a great baby. After a quick change from dairy to soya milk, she settled really well into feeding and sleeping. She ate and slept for those precious first few weeks, and I fell head over heels in love with her. That said, I was still extremely traumatised after Keri's birth, and it featured in my nurturing of Lucy. I obsessed over Lucy's breathing, always so terrified she would die by cot death. I persistently checked that she was alive. I was so hypervigilant that I purchased a baby monitor with a camera and a small TV unit so I could keep a close watch on her at all times, both by day and by night.

Between caring for Keri and my close surveillance of Lucy, sleep did not feature in my life at this time. My days and nights were fueled by caffeine, love, and determination. I need not have worried about Lucy. She fell into a great routine and thrived as the gorgeous little lady she was and the gorgeous young lady she is now. Although her big sister was a brunette, Lucy similarly had the most gorgeous blonde ringlet curls and a smile that would light up the world. Our world was complete once Lucy came along.

After a really successful 'bonus year' in pre-school, Keri was now more than ready to start Primary School in September 2009. At this stage, Keri was one month off her 6th birthday. I was so pleased that we held her back. It gave her every chance of success in the 'big school' and successful it was.

Scoil Aoughusa is a co-educational (girls and boys) school in Cashel, Co Tipperary, for students with learning disabilities. The school nurtures each child as an individual and adapts the curriculum to meet his/her specific needs. Its mission is 'Developing Ability – Diminishing Disability.' Students in Scoil Aonghusa participate in many activities, and they are actively involved in Special Olympics, which Keri would later hugely enjoy. Keri was blessed with her place there, in the exceptional care of her Nurses Catherine and Geraldine, together with the team under Principal Siobhan.

Keri had a lot in common with Siobhan - both absolutely loved their style. Every day, without fail, Siobhan would make it her business to meet Keri during the day and marvel at her style. Keri really enjoyed her grand entrance each morning to her classroom, decked out in the brightest of colours, and she lapped up all the compliments. Keri was never a girl for the darkness. She loved big, bright, bold colours-pinks, purples, oranges and reds, together with the obligatory sparkles wherever possible! How fitting it was for Keri's classroom to be the 'rainbow room', where she settled so happily, reunited with her boyfriend from preschool, James Cooney.

Keri's wellbeing was central to everything at Scoil Aoughusa as she settled into school. The rainbow room always had a Nurse assigned to it, and Keri was so very well looked after. Over the years, Keri came under the care of exceptional teachers, therapists and carers, always full of cheer with such incredible kindness. When her health allowed it, she commuted to and from school by bus with her friend Tamara, driven by Haulie, Brendan, Robert, Michael, Andy or Larry. These gentlemen were always so welcoming and incredibly careful in bringing Keri and her friends to and from school.

9

Truth

On the 7th of March, 2007, the HSE filed a full defence to Keri's case. They admitted nothing, and they denied everything. The battle was on. An affidavit of verification, a sworn document signed on oath to confirm the truth to the defence, was filed. Our home and livelihoods were at risk, and the HSE were staring us down. This was heating up to be ruthless litigation. We had done none of the wrongdoing but were living with all the risk and dire consequences.

On receiving the Defence, our solicitor wrote to the HSE seeking discovery of documents (where important documents relevant to a dispute are sought as part of the court process), including the report which should have been drawn up after Keri's birth was investigated. This report was denied to us under the Freedom of Information Act. The HSE denied that we were entitled to these documents. The HSE argued that they were legally 'privileged'. Keri was certainly not living a life of 'privilege' thanks to their negligence. Our lawyers sought an order in the Master's Court. We lost that battle. The decision was appealed to the High Court. This was successful, and finally, after a protracted battle, we were granted access to the internal investigation report.

It was at that stage (three years later) that I learned, to my horror, that, in July 2004, nine months after Keri's birth, the HSE knew of significant systems failures in this case. Significant clinical risk management concerns were identified in the report regarding failures in training and competency of staff, and most horrifyingly, training in respect of CTG monitoring. This report was 'Red Flagged' and deliberately buried and obstructed by the HSE until such time as a High Court Order pushed its release some three years later. During that time and knowing of these 'significant concerns', a full defence to our claim for Keri's brain injury was put up. Due to their incompetence during Keri's birth, the HSE created our nightmare. In their belligerence, they intensified it with this appalling mishandling of our data and blocking Keri's information and access to justice.

Over those three years since the report was issued (and the HSE knew of the wrongs done), we were left to our own devices without the support she deserved. Keri missed out on so much neuro-rehabilitation that we simply could not financially afford for her. Time is of the essence in cases like this-years lost without rehabilitation is an opportunity gone forever. Motor skills, like rolling over, crawling or sitting unaided, not learned in infancy, cannot later be mastered. Early intervention is key. Keri never mastered those skills, as we relied on public services (amazing staff, inadequate resources) and whatever I could buy with the proceeds from my childminding hours.

The report from the Paediatric Neurologist was returned. It confirmed our very worst nightmare, printed in black and white. Prior to my labour, Keri was a perfectly healthy, full-term baby. She had no pre-existing issues or ailments. It was the barbaric management of my labour and her too-late delivery which had plainly caused her avoidable, but now irreversible, catastrophic brain damage. To add salt to the now re-opened wounds, we also learned that the negligence didn't even stop there. After Keri was delivered, strangled by the cord, she was almost dead. She required invasive resuscitation (not just a mask) to bring her little body and brain back to life. The team in Kilkenny could not assemble the apparatus to intubate her. They couldn't manage it, not knowing what to do. It was not for many more hours that she was intubated by the neonatal team who came from Waterford. The brain damaging negligence continued, even after she was born. As was described in Court some years later, Keri suffered 'insult, heaped upon injury.'

Our final medical report to prove the responsibility of the hospital was from a paediatric neuro-radiologist, who examined Keri's MRI and confirmed the pattern of her brain injury was in line with that described by the neurologist and not from any other cause. That report confirmed and finalised the evidence from a fault perspective. There was no other reason for Keri's disability. We had now proven our case that Keri was brain damaged at birth from Gross Medical Negligence, an injury that was entirely avoidable if I was in the right hands during my labour. It was now for us to take on the HSE and battle to prove it in Court.

At the time the reports were issued, and revisiting them now in writing this book, I am still not angry. The reason I hold no anger is because Keri lived. That said, to this day, I am still in complete dismay that the staff in question didn't simply put their hands up and say that they were in over their heads. As a result, Keri suffered enormously. My distress lies with Keri's lifetime of suffering. Ever since my labour commenced, that suffering never ended until she took her last breath.

My subconscious self sometimes wonders, as a mother, was I protecting Keri as I should have? Could I have shouted louder? Would that have made a difference? I will live with this question for the rest of my life. If hindsight is to teach us anything from this story, I would say as mothers, we have to go with our gut. All the information is with our instinct. It shouldn't be dismissed by ourselves or by anyone else. We should not presume that the best way to be is 'polite' or 'ladylike'; we must speak up as to what we are feeling. That said, it was a relief to have confirmation from the experts that it wasn't my fault. Armed with those reports, my logical mind knew that what occurred was a series of errors which had no connection with my management of things.

My predominant feeling at this stage was that HSE simply had to own up to what they had done wrong, both for Keri and for other families. Although it was awful news, it felt good to know that we were right to risk it all for Keri to have justice. The more reports that returned in support of her case, the more ablaze the fire in my belly became to fight for Keri so she would have justice done and the best life possible in her predicament. I was never going to let this go unless I got an admission of liability and an apology. That was my primary goal for Keri. It meant nothing that this 'wasn't something the HSE normally do'. Keri was not going to be simply paid off to go away. From that day onwards, I never second guessed myself on the court case. I knew I had got this piece right. I was going to see it through to the just and proper end.

10

Contentment

Our noisy, crazy lives at home continued with the gorgeous company of my own girls, Kate, Carrie, Jack and Emily. I had also been looking after sisters Amy and Sophie O'Brien for two years. Laughter was always our very best medicine, and we were blessed to be bathed in it with the children I was so privileged to look after. One of the funniest memories I have was a particular afternoon when Kate, Carrie, Jack, Emily, Sophie and Lucy were in the garden, playing on the trampoline. I was standing at the sink looking out at them. All of a sudden, Lucy jumped and disappeared out of sight. She had jumped straight through a hole in the trampoline and disappeared! I collapsed in a heap laughing. The expressions on all their faces are one that has never left my memory. Eventually, I did pull myself together enough to go out and check if she was OK, which thankfully she was, laughing her little head off. We still laugh about that incident to this day.

In 2007, unwavering in gratitude for the help Keri was receiving from the Jack and Jill Foundation, we decided to organise a second Valentine's fundraiser ball, which took place on the 16th of February, 2008. This event also supported the Brothers of Charity, who had been so good to us in the provision of education for Keri at *Lus na Greine*. This was a more difficult fundraiser to get over the line. The *Celtic Tiger* was dying fast, and cash had become scarce to come by. I brought Keri along to the event this time. Her health was up to it, and I knew she and the guests would enjoy her being there, as transpired to be the case. She lit up the room and was met with such warmth from those who met her, some for the very first time. Thanks to all the generosity of the people of Fethard and surrounding areas, together with our Keri as the star of the night, we managed to raise almost €40,000.

Keri's teeth continued to cause her trouble. Unfortunately, eight had to be extracted in 2008, when Keri was five years old, based on a review by the paediatric dentist in Dublin. Two molars, left and right, top and bottom, had to be removed. The essential medication had inevitably caused further extensive tooth decay. Following the extractions, Keri developed a nasty gum infection, which required hospitalisation and IV antibiotics for a number of days. Nothing was easy for poor Keri, but she battled through and recovered, giving us back her enchanting smile as soon as she possibly could.

The contentment of a walk with the girls, seeing them smile and enjoying time together, was all the nourishment I needed. We often went for a walk and a take-away coffee got chocolate buttons for Keri and whatever treat Lucy picked out, and we would sit on the wall across from the ballroom, enjoy our treats, and walk and wheel home. The most simple, profound joy was in those moments with my two girls.

Keri graduated from *Lus na Greine* preschool on the 23rd of July, 2009. It was such an incredibly proud and emotional day for us all. Keri had been through so much, but she had fought every battle to take her rightful place in the world and to prosper. At *Lus na Greine*, Keri and her community of wonderful friends were like little sunflowers, and they had blossomed in the light of an exceptional team that had brought out the very best in them all. The book of photographs and memories of all of Keri's fun, laughter and learning in *Lus na Greine* will always be treasured, and her time there will always hold a special place in my heart.

The summer of 2009 was a flurry of appointments with experts retained to give evidence in Court on Keri's requirements. Now that we had established wrongdoing, we had to establish, with expert evidence, what was required to make life as comfortable as possible for Keri. Following consultations and examinations in each field, reports were taken up from a Physiotherapist, Occupational Therapist, Speech and Language Therapist, Nursing Care expert, Vocational expert, Engineer and Actuary. It required a huge commitment and thousands of miles driving to attend each of these meetings, not only to build our own case but on the demands of the HSE experts who also looked to examine Keri and consider her position from a defence perspective.

For every report we retained, the HSE countered it. I found that so difficult. I sometimes got angry that the HSE would keep dragging an innocent child through all these appointments, especially when they knew all along what they did and could have done the right thing far earlier. That part broke my heart-it was more needless suffering for Keri. She was entitled to object to such a gruelling schedule of examinations, but true to form and good as gold, she put her best smile on and charmed them all with her disarming smile.

The run-up to the Court hearing was an incredibly stressful time for Chalkie, Lucy and I. I will never forget on the eve of one appointment we had to attend with Keri in the UK, Lucy, who was only two years of age at the time, had an accident at home and pulled a cup of hot tea onto herself, which landed her in the emergency department. The following morning, Chalkie, Keri, Lucy, and I still had to travel. Regardless of the circumstances, we had to fight on. We had no choice. Domestic difficulties, even in a family like ours, are not a consideration in the gruelling Court process.

11

Admission

The day when everything changed, and yet absolutely nothing changed, was the 29th of July, 2009. It was the regular midweek routine. I had been caring for Lucy and the other six children at home while Keri was at school. That afternoon, Keri and I were driving to Clonmel to see her Osteopath. Susie Elliott, a Solicitor at Cantillons, telephoned me. I told her that we were on the road to Clonmel for Keri's appointment. Susie requested that I pull into the side of the road. I did as I was told. Before she spoke further, she checked that the car was parked.

'Clodagh, I have a letter here that you will be keen to hear of. It has just arrived by fax. It is a letter from Hayes Solicitors, who have taken over the defence of your case against the HSE. This is an important letter. It confirms that the HSE has admitted liability. They have accepted responsibility for Keri's injuries. Keri has won her case.' She paused. I burst into tears. 'I am sorry for you all that the wrong occurred, but justice has finally been done. All that remains now is for the case to be argued on quantum, that is, damages or money, how much the HSE are liable to pay to compensate Keri for her injuries.'

I had no words for Susie. I was relieved all at once. My precious Keri was now only weeks away from her 6th birthday. This admission of liability should have happened before I even took her home from the hospital. The HSE knew, many years ago, that there was a problem with the management of Keri's birth. Yet it had taken 6 years to admit it. That delay wasn't just stressful, costly and unnecessary. It cost Keri a rehabilitation opportunity that she never could get back. For Keri, justice was delayed, and therefore justice was denied.

The admission of liability meant that our family home and financial future were no longer at risk, but I was so hurt that it had taken so long. For Keri's first 6 years, we simply could not afford to buy her all the treatments, therapies, equipment and help she so desperately needed. Chalkie was working hard, and I was now minding 6 children in addition to my own two just to make ends meet. We were exhausted and had little help from the state. I fuelled my days and nights with caffeine, yet there were days when I hadn't the price of a coffee in my purse. While I always did my best for Keri, it simply was not possible to give her all she required. This lack, this deficit in care and rehabilitation, cost Keri enormously, and it cost her permanently. The HSE therapists are incredible, they did all they could, but resources are so limited within the system that Keri needed her public service supplemented privately.

We couldn't afford this, so she never got, for example, the level of Physiotherapy she required, thereby losing her ability to roll over, her potential to crawl, and her ability to hold her head in prone. She began to develop contractures. She regressed in her motor skills. Her spine had started to curve. All those developmental milestones and so much potential to have been physically stronger were lost forever simply because of a criminal failure by the HSE to do the right thing, to admit the wrongdoing, to compensate Keri quickly and to give her the best chance at life possible.

Further 'insult heaped on injury' arose when the lawyers started to debate Keri's Life Expectancy. In cases like Keri's, which are termed 'catastrophic injury cases', the question of how long a Plaintiff is expected to live becomes a central point of contention. In Keri's case, the HSE had (too late in the day) admitted liability. That meant that we no longer had to argue the facts of her birth in Court to establish wrongdoing. What was left to be argued, however, was the question of quantum-as Susie had explained, how much the HSE were liable to pay. To date, despite acres of work by various legal groups, cases like this are still concluded on a 'lump sum' basis. These cases are complete with a once-off, full and final payment.

This lump sum must suffice for the entirety of the Plaintiff's life. But how long will any of us live? Nobody knows, but in cases like Keri's, various factors are considered by the experts, like, for example, the ability to feed independently without aspiration, lift the head in prone, roll over, crawl, and walk. In Keri's case, it was those very factors, lost on Keri because of the delay in getting justice, that the HSE flagged in their favour to seek to avoid payment for further years they argued she wouldn't have.

I had to park the emotions these letters, timelines and reports had stirred up in me. I had 8 children to mind and a court case to prepare for. Keri had lived. There was still no anger. I held no bitterness. I was making this work as I promised I would. Mug of coffee in hand, game face on. We marched on together.

12

Vindication

I learned, in October 2009, that the High Court is no place of joy. It is a large, grey, cemented structure on the dusty, rumbling quays of Dublin city centre. It is peppered with a multitude of heavy creaking doors, swished through by wigged, robed lawyers, holding for the person coming after with a polite but rushed nod. It is a place of cold, tiled, narrow corridors cobbled with lawyers in huddled gatherings and whisperings, the lay clients so easily identifiable by their petrified expressions. It is a place where even the hardiest of stomachs will succumb to the nerves, in the bowels of the 'round hall' blue-lamped toilets, burst open the bowels of Plaintiffs like me, Mum of a brain damaged child, fighting for her baby.

The practical arrangements for attending Court were enormous. Caitriona sourced alternative childcare. Chalkie took time off work to take care of Keri and Lucy, with Cora rowing in for further hours, while I attended in Dublin. Mammy travelled with me each morning, departing home at 6am to take the train from Thurles to

Heuston Station Dublin, returning home after 9pm at night.

It was mentally and physically draining, but I am good under pressure, especially when fighting for my children. In this case, I was Keri's voice, and I simply could not let her down. I was nervous but hugely focused. I wanted Keri's story to be told. I wanted the world to hear that she had fought so hard to get to her 6th birthday, which we had only celebrated the day before, that each day had brought both good and bad challenges and that I accepted each and every one with all my heart, grateful that she had survived and that I had the privilege to be her mother.

After going over so many gruelling medico-legal reports, I wanted the record straight that although Keri had severe disabilities, she was a gift, not a hindrance, and she had brought so much beauty and love to the world. If her most intimate details were to be aired, then I wanted to bring her pinks, her purples, her sparkles and her deep love to the cold walls of the Four Courts. Keri, as she always did, was going to bring light to this heartless legal system. I would make sure of it.

Navigating such an inhumane legal system in such a heartless building, Keri was blessed with the most wonderful legal team. Solicitors Ernest Cantillon and Susie Elliott prepared the case seamlessly and submitted it to Senior Counsel Liam Reidy and Oonah McCrann, together with Junior Counsel John Lucey, for presentation to the Court. These five lawyers were down to earth but highly skilled and experienced. They did a remarkable job of making us feel comfortable and at ease, so we could, as a unified team, ensure the best job was done for Keri.

I have clear memories of Ernest, one of Ireland's most senior Solicitors, pouring us tea during a consultation, offering around biscuits, all the while watching every move of the team, making sure not a trick was missed. Oonah, an extraordinary lawyer, a wife, a woman and a mother herself, related to me so openly. She carefully and skillfully took me through my evidence in Court, examining my case in her questioning with both compassion and razor-sharp precision. Liam, a bright, witty, genuine man of enormous experience, opened our case with the most damning, poignant, powerful speech, condemning the HSE for its brinkmanship in defending Keri's case for so long. John, who had been involved in the case since commencement, proved a wise, industrious, and genuinely helpful barrister at every turn. Susie walked the path with me through so many years, before, during and after this Court case. She was there for us in all our ups and downs and has transformed from being our lawyer to one of our very special friends.

The meetings in 'Consultation Room 8A' were far from easy. The question of how long my cherished baby would live became the base upon which the calculations were made. In simple terms, how much measure could be put on Keri's lifespan, and how much money would it take for the HSE to see her off from this litigation?

For us, Keri deserved the best of everything, which, if provided, would hugely increase her life expectancy. For the HSE, Keri was entitled only to what their experts had sparingly listed in confusing and illogical reports which were drafted to save the State money. The HSE argued that Keri's lifespan was short, arising from unreached milestones. One harrowing HSE report detailed how Keri's spine would mercilessly curve and twist, ultimately destroying her lung and stomach function, causing pneumonia and bowel failure, which would signal the end of her short life. Meanwhile, our reports set out all that she could achieve if afforded the best of care, therapies and equipment.

It was the most heart wrenching battle. I clearly recall explaining to Liam Reidy in room 8A my sincere, heartfelt wish at the time, which was, 'If God has any mercy at all, he will take Keri before me because I know that only I can do the very best for her. Nobody will love and care for her like I do.' A mother never wants to lose her child to death, but given Keri's condition, my wish was that I would see out her every moment so that her every day would be the best possible day and inhale life to its fullest moment until that time came.

The court hearing began on Wednesday, 21st October, 2009. Adrenaline and caffeine coursed through my veins. Liam told me that a measly and insulting offer had been made by the HSE to settle the case, which he had refused on my behalf. The hearing commenced before Mr Justice Lavan.

Liam's opening speech was harrowing. He described in detail every relevant part of Keri's journey into and through the world following her brutal start to life. He portrayed the maneuvering by the HSE in defence of this case. He explained how, in spite of the (belated) admission of liability, the HSE still didn't have the decency to explain what had gone wrong or why an admission had taken so long to be forthcoming. He noted the apology by the HSE was only given after it had been called for by Keri's lawyers, saying that a sought for apology is no apology at all. He went on to describe Keri's condition and requirements in detail. A video of Keri at home had been prepared, which was played for the judge so he could understand Keri's needs and capabilities. It was clear at the end of Liam's opening speech that Keri was a child with an enormous disability who would require round-the-clock care for the rest of her life. Liam's opening took up the entire first day. He did an incredible job to advocate for my Keri. I was relieved to be in such good hands.

Day two was my day to give evidence. As the Court resumed, Mr Justice Lavan immediately requested details as to the sums being claimed in Keri's case, to which Oonah gave detailed costings. It was apparent to me that the judge had heard enough, in this case where liability had been admitted, to encourage the parties to negotiate a settlement, if at all possible. Protracted legal battles serve nobody, not least the two little girls at home in Tipperary without their mother for all those long days. Both sides were encouraged to engage in discussions.

I was incredibly nervous before taking the stand, so much so that I suffered an upset stomach and almost had a panic attack outside the Courtroom. I knew I had to settle down and do the best for Keri. Susie advised that I look at the judge at all times while answering the questions put to me and forget about everyone else in the Courtroom. Once I started and proceeded with that technique, I settled in well and developed a great rapport with the judge. I wanted him to see the bigger picture, see the child, not just the disability or the litigation. Keri was the light of my life, and my evidence had to allow everyone to see the beauty in her, what she could do and not just what she couldn't do. I felt the HSE wanted to put her down at every turn of this case. There was an injustice to that, too, that I wanted to correct. The point for me was to give Keri the better life she deserved, to allow her to blossom into her best self.

Oonah questioned me for my 'evidence in chief'. She was incredibly gentle yet highly skilled in her craft, ensuring the judge had the full picture of my background, our marriage, our home, our prior miscarriage, our pregnancy, my labour and Keri's delivery. She brought me through all the details of Keri's early years, her slow progress with milestones, her excruciating spasms, feeding strategies and the various therapies we employed to help her. I was at pains to explain to the judge that a PEG feeding regime, while it may be easier and 'cheaper' for the HSE to pay for, was not best for Keri, who really enjoyed her meals. I was anxious to point out that it was what was best for Keri that was most important, not what was easier or less expensive to implement. Every moment of Keri's day and night was covered by Oonah's questioning. Keri's complete life story was told. Judge Lavan was a lovely man who made me feel very at ease in answering Oonah's questions. I subsequently heard from our Counsel that the judge was visibly intrigued by my descriptions with gestures of the energy work that is inherent in some of Keri's alternative therapies-material never before put before the Courts in Ireland! I was proud that Keri was, once again, breaking new ground in the world, shining a light on new and sometimes better ways to manage things.

A Consultant Paediatrician who had examined Keri on our side was then called to give evidence questioned by Liam. This doctor had examined Keri in the UK in November 2008 for the purpose of submitting a current condition and prognosis report to the court. His evidence was in relation to what Keri needed and would need for her future, estimating, as best he could, how long that future would be. The testimony was well delivered, and I was very pleased with the elements of Keri's personality and preference that were celebrated by both the barrister and the doctor. Keri had a way of bringing out the best in people, and I saw only the very best in these professionals at that moment. Keri's preferences for stories, music and her awareness of her surroundings - the things that matter most, were all covered.

Life expectancy was then discussed in detail. There was no avoiding it. I was very pleased to learn that the central root of life expectancy was argued to be around the quality of care; something I would ensure would never be compromised for Keri. I knew that was an element I certainly could control! Evidence of the Paediatrician continued the following day. A coordinated symphony of Physiotherapy, Occupational Therapy, Speech Therapy, Botox, Hydrotherapy, appropriate Housing and Nursing Care were all argued for. I felt we were chipping away at a victory for Keri, for her to get all the comfort and care she so truly deserved. I knew she had stolen every heart in that courtroom, no matter which side of the battle they were on. The Court adjourned for lunch.

Negotiations continued. Various offers were made. It all came down to how much money was required to care for Keri each year and how many years she was likely to live. It was a gruelling, stressful, scary process. In the end, it was down to me, as Keri's legal next friend, to decide if the 'final offer' would be sufficient to look after Keri for the whole of her life, however long that would be. The final lump sum settlement would never be the correct sum. The only correct sum would be that the last euro is spent on the last moment of life. This could never be calculated. It was only ever going to be too much or too little, and it was never going to compensate Keri for the pain and distress she had suffered and would suffer every moment of her precious life. Once the final lump sum figure of €4.5

million was reached in the hands of such educated and skilled professionals who recommended it, I accepted this offer on Keri's behalf.

As Keri was a minor, her settlement had to be 'ruled' or approved by another High Court judge. The hearing was adjourned to allow this to happen. When it resumed, Chalkie and I brought Keri to Court. I wanted to introduce her to her legal team and bring her sparkle to the dark, soulless Four Courts complex. In Court, I was again asked to explain our circumstances and to indicate my level of satisfaction with the settlement offer. The media were in attendance for this hearing. What was most important to me was that the letter of apology, which had been sent to our solicitors earlier that month, be read in Court. It meant nothing unless it was read out loud for all the world to hear so that my little girl could be publicly vindicated. The judge approved the settlement offer and praised us for all our work for Keri since her birth. Counsel for the HSE read the apology out loud before the Court and media as follows:

'We have taken our client's instructions on this matter and, in light of the fact that liability is now admitted, our client is more than happy to offer a full and unreserved apology to all of the plaintiffs herein for its acts and/or omissions in relation to its management of Clodagh Brett's labour and the delivery of Keri Brett. A full and unreserved apology is offered by both the Health Service Executive and St Luke's General Hospital Kilkenny in relation to the matters pleaded

in the Personal Injuries summons and in relation to the undoubted trauma which has been suffered by all the plaintiffs herein as a result thereof.'

We eventually received the apology we had sought six years earlier. Chalkie and I wheeled our incredible little girl with all her sparkles out to the gates of the Four Courts. I addressed the media, calling for a medical duty of candour, calling for doctors to be legally obliged to explain what went wrong and why it went wrong when a harmful medical event occurs. We called for protracted litigation in cases like this to stop, as it was causing real and permanent damage. The week that followed was a busy one, with a flurry of media interviews, but I was happy to do it. I didn't want another injured child to suffer like Keri did at the hands of the HSE.

To this day, I strongly believe that the swifter approach by the HSE we now see in Medical Negligence cases comes down to Keri's fight and example as to how these matters should properly be handled. I have since referred plenty of families to our legal team, and many a happy ending has flowed from these referrals. Keri brought out the best in her lawyers, as indeed, she did in all her exchanges.

13

Neighbourhood

Funds for Keri, which flowed from the Court case, were paid by the State Claims Agency to Keri's account in the Office of the Wards of Court. This is an office overseen by the President of the High Court where funds and activities of minors (those under 18 years of age) and adults without capacity are handled. In Keri's case, she became a Minor Ward of the Court, so her funds were held and managed by this office of the High Court. Keri was assigned a case officer who expertly coordinated and arranged payments to fund her care and equipment following sign off by the President of the High Court. The Court was so careful with Keri's funds and very particular to ensure they were put to best use. It gave me great comfort to know that I didn't have to manage Keri's money, which had to fund her every need for the rest of her life. I had enough to be worrying about. By then, addressing Keri's housing requirements was beyond overdue.

Chalkie and I built our first house together, a modest but gorgeous 3-bedroom bungalow in Fethard in 1997.

I was only twenty one years old at the time. We were so proud to own our own home as such a young couple. For the first seven years of her life, this was Keri's home, too, but it was totally unsuited to her needs. When the house was constructed, there were no legal regulations requiring wheelchair accessibility in private homes. As a young, carefree couple, such accessibility didn't occur to us.

In the early days of Keri's life, we invested in a cement ramp to the front entrance of the house. This was the only useful part of the house for Keri and, indeed, her only access. There were steps at the back and conservatory doors, so those access points were out of bounds for her. Internally, the house was not accessible. The hall was too narrow to turn a wheelchair, and one had to come to the top of the hall and turn the chair in order to come back down in the opposite direction. With Keri's wheelchair in the sitting room with the sofa and two armchairs, there wasn't much room for manoeuvre.

None of the bedrooms were wheelchair accessible. At the time, Keri was in a small chair, but I could barely squeeze it in. I couldn't wheel her around any of the rooms. One of the bedrooms was used purely for her equipment, but to take out one item, all items had to be unloaded to access it. Once the required item was retrieved, all other items would have to be put back. We packed and unpacked that room multiple times a day. Nothing was simple. The kitchen was very tight.

Bathing Keri in our tiny bathroom was a difficult and oftentimes dangerous task. With so little space to manoeuvre, I bathed Keri in a specialised chair in the bath, afterwards transferring her onto a towel placed on the floor. After her bath, I would carefully (and awkwardly) lift her out of the bath and place her down on the ground, wrap her up as fast as possible, lift her off the floor and quickly carry her out to the bedroom to dry her off and dress her as Keri got cold so quickly.

On two particular occasions, whilst lifting Keri off the floor, I slipped on the wet bathroom tiles and cracked my head off the toilet bowl. Luckily, on both occasions, I managed to protect Keri from injury, but I was terrified that if I had been knocked unconscious, what would have happened to Keri? After those two dangerous incidents, I always made sure that there was someone else in the house when I was bathing her.

After the second fall, OT Joanne organised another specialized chair, a replica of what was in the bath, but it was at hip level and on wheels, which was known as a shower tray to place Keri onto after her bath, rather than the floor. With this chair, I was able to keep Keri off the floor, up at my level, preventing any further such accidents. This was an extra piece of equipment in our house that we had no space for, but it was a necessity.

But for Keri's disabilities, it would have been a perfect home for the four of us. While historically, I absolutely loved this home and was so proud of it, after Keri arrived, it became only bricks and mortar. For me, Keri's welfare, comfort and safety were all that mattered.

In considering a wish list for Keri's new home, I was very clear on what she liked, disliked and required from a comfort, practicality, and safety perspective. While we initially considered building an extension to our original bungalow, it soon became apparent that there was not sufficient land to cater for Keri's needs. During the course of the Court Case, Keri's solicitors retained the services of Fiana Barry, Occupational Therapist and Tony O Keeffe, Engineer, both highly experienced professionals in the area of special needs provision. Tony and Fiana's respective reports allowed afforded us an opportunity to learn what was out there, what might work best for Keri and what sort of facilities she would need.

I retained the services of Mark Collins and Stephen Brennan of CBA Architecture to assist us. Although there was a family connection between Stephen and I, it was made perfectly clear from the outset that this was a formal business relationship, and it proceeded as such from day one. Mark, Stephen and I carefully went through all of Keri's requirements and set to work to find a feasible solution. Mark and Stephen did an exemplary job and certainly kept their side of the bargain.

We commenced our search for a site to build upon. This was not easy. We looked at countless pockets of land, but Planning Permission and location constraints made it extremely tricky. I contacted John Stokes, a local auctioneer from Fethard with an office in Clonmel. I explained our circumstances and asked for his help. John obliged wholeheartedly and went to great lengths to find a solution for us. He contacted a lady who owned land in Garrinch on the outskirts of Fethard, and she agreed to sell us an acre. We never met this lady; John looked after everything and made it so easy for us. I was brought to see a flat site, which I had indicated was important for Keri's access.

The site is conveniently located close to Fethard town in a peaceful, private countryside location. Horses graze in a neighbouring field to the east, and to the northeast, one's eyes are drawn to the rooftops of Fethard with its enchanting backdrop, Slievenamon mountains, decorated with acres of forestry, snowcapped in winter, teeming with new life in spring. Garrinch is a neighbourhood of old. On one occasion, we met a gentleman by the name of Sham, who was born and reared in the same house that he continues to reside to this day, who very kindly gave us such a beautiful run down of how special this neighbourhood was, one which people do not leave. Families grow and are nourished here. This is what I wanted for my girls. We were absolutely overjoyed when the sale went through on this very special site in the company of such welcoming neighbours.

In early 2010, not long after the Court case concluded, we received very upsetting news. Marty Davey was let go from work; therefore, understandably, I was no longer required as their formal childminder. I was devastated, the Davey kids were devastated as they had become part of our family, and we were all so contented with our busy, noisy lives together. Thankfully, to this day, the Davey family still are very much part of our family. They call weekly and have regular sleepovers. They are a massive part of our lives and always will be. They refer to me as their adopted Mammy, a title I am very proud of! It means the world to me, and I agree wholeheartedly when the Davey family tell me that they would not be the (fabulous) people they are today were it not for having Keri in their lives. They never took things for granted, as they saw the struggle Keri endured to do simple tasks like roll over. Keri taught us all so much. If it were not for Keri, I would never have been their childminder. Once again, Keri blessed all of us.

14

Spasms

While the search for Keri's new home was underway, her spasms massively escalated in 2010. They became relentless, just like back in the very early days. They were taking over her life again. It was a really difficult situation to manage. During one particular week, I had to go to school to collect her on a number of days, such was her distress. While the spasms were always a problem for Keri, they became manageable for a period until 2010, when Keri's condition deteriorated at the age of seven. The doctors reviewed all her medications. Baclofen, also known as Lioresal, was increased on a number of occasions, specifically to help manage the spasms.

Being the inquisitive, determined type of mother I am, I started journaling the medication and noting the side effects. In particular, I questioned the Baclofen because, to my surprise, I read that one of the side effects of this medication (to treat spasms) is an increase in spasms. I brought this up at various medical appointments but was assured this would be most unlikely the cause of

Keri's increasing spasms. The brutal suffering went on and on, and the spasms got worse and worse. I was so frustrated and upset for Keri. My suggestion to take Keri off Baclofen was not entertained by them, as there was no available alternative. The Baclofen was increased repeatedly. I watched carefully for a few days, but there was only a further marked deterioration.

To describe a spasm for Keri is to describe a form of immense, extended, brutal and unexplainable torture experienced by an innocent disabled child who doesn't understand what is happening to her little body. The episodes appeared like seizures, but they were spasms – painful contractions of every muscle in her body caused by neurological disruption arising from her brain injury.

A spasm would start with her arms extending and shaking her whole body, then work up to an outright prolonged stiff shudder with her face turning purple. During this time, Keri would gasp for her every breath, absolutely terrified. She would wail, and the fear in her face would shatter my heart as the spasms and waves of agony would come again and again, overcoming her, torturing her, terrifying her.

On the bad days, Keri would have no reprieve before another spasm would overcome her. If Keri was having a mild spasm, I would catch her quickly with a tight embrace, and it may only last a minute, but as things got worse in 2010, the spasms could last up to 4 minutes of the most horrific, terrifying, uncontrollable pain.

After the spasm, she would be exhausted and need a lot of comfort and cuddles. I will never forget her petrified little face when she had these spasms. The cruelty of it was that Keri never got used to them, no matter how many she experienced. The first was as scary as the fiftieth that she may have in one day. Every spasm was a brand new, brutal and terrifying trauma.

At the worst point in this period, Keri was suffering episodes every 15 minutes of the entire day. She would barely come out of one spasm before another would start. Keri was so unwell that I asked Cora to look after Lucy instead of Keri, as I simply could not be away from her at this time. She would scream her little heart out after each spasm, and all I could do was wrap my arms around her as tight as I could to try and comfort her. Although I continued to give it, Buccal Midazolam (a benzodiazepine medication used to treat conditions including seizures and Spasms) just wasn't helping her any more.

Enough was enough. This endless, relentless, compounding suffering had gone on for months, and there was no more anyone could do. Everyone had run out of ideas, but it wasn't for the want of trying by her medical team. Keri was in non-stop agony and terror. Her life was hardly worth living. I worried that her little heart could no longer take it, and this was confirmed by a doctor as a real possibility. I decided that I would take Keri off Baclofen myself. I told nobody. I knew what my gut was telling me, and I just had to go with it. By secretly taking

Keri off Baclofen, no medical professional would be part of any controversy that might arise.

Three weeks of hell ensued. The vicious spasms continued, and she suffered terrible withdrawals from the Baclofen. However, as time went on, I could see an improvement in Keri. Her spasm frequency dropped from about fifty to ten a day, which made life worth living again.

Once I had Keri off the Baclofen and out of the withdrawals, I told the doctors what I had done. Surprisingly, they were supportive but understandably anxious to work on further medical solutions to the ongoing spasms. Various medications from the *pam* family were trialed-diazepam, clonazepam, etc., but none of them agreed with Keri.

Eventually, it was suggested that Keri would be brought to Beaumont Hospital to have the IBT (Intrathecal Balcofen Therapy) clinic carry out tests to see if a Balcofen pump could be inserted into Keri's body. I could not understand why this was considered a good idea. Keri had been off Balcofen for some time now, and the spasm activity had hugely decreased as a result. I didn't see the logic in putting her back on it, albeit by a different route. I argued my case as hard as I could, but I lost the battle. Against my better judgment, Keri was admitted to have the IBT trial. I was so upset. I knew this was a bad idea. The IBT protocol involves the initial insertion of an external Baclofen pump to see if it is successful, following which, if successful, an internal pump is fitted for ongoing internal administration of the drug. I tried to explain to the medical team once again that Keri was previously on Baclofen, that the spasms had increased with each increase in dosage and that I had withdrawn her from it, successfully reducing her spasms. Nobody listened. I was put into a position whereby I had no choice but to consent to the procedure, as I was told nothing more could or would be done for Keri if I refused this one. It was made very clear to me that I am not a medical professional, and therefore, my opinion on this proposed treatment didn't count. It was so difficult because I knew first-hand how much Keri had gone through to come off the Baclofen, and now they wanted to pump it into her! It was a nightmare.

I wished they had listened to me that day in June 2011 and all the other days I had made a logical case against this drug. At one stage, I was told, 'I did not spend all these years to become a doctor for you tell me what you think is wrong with your child. I am the doctor, not you'. I had pleaded for them not to do it, but I was silenced. Following the insertion of the trial pump, Keri returned from the theatre in a horrendous state, suffering the most unthinkable muscle spasms. I was so cross and so upset I called for the doctor to attend immediately, and when she came, she could not believe her eyes. 'Look at the pain you have caused Keri. I was made to do this to my child, and none of you would listen to me'. The IBT pump and lead were quickly removed. She was then given medication to counteract the dreadful spasms she was suffering. It took Keri countless hours to settle again after this. It was absolutely dreadful to be ignored and dismissed as I was in relation to that procedure, and it caused incredible terror, pain and distress to Keri, which was totally avoidable.

When it came to my precious Keri, I was not going to be shoved to the side ever again. This experience made my lioness mom's voice roar louder for the years ahead. I was reminded of the late Dr Eddie McGrath's advice to his junior doctor colleagues to always listen to the parents, as they know their child best. I don't think any of the doctors who forced that procedure on Keri were blessed with a training under Dr McGrath. I have no medical degree, but I had lived with Keri's condition twenty-four hours a day to that point, some eight years at that stage. I wasn't long learning all there was to know-I had no choice-I was left to sink or swim. Frankly, a lot of the knowledge I have gathered is common sense, but I have learned along the way that common sense is not so common.

Keri and I did receive an apology for the IBT incident. The doctor felt bad for what happened and did all she could to help, including prescribing Zanaflex (Tizanidine), which helped massively with Keri's spasticity. This helped Keri hugely and allowed her to relax sufficiently to sleep somewhat better at night. In the end, that doctor did a lot of good for Keri, and I hold no resentment. She gave a lot of time trying to come up with an alternative to Baclofen, and she dug deep. Thanks to her, Keri got great relief from this new medication, which she took going forward. It was a learning point for everyone. I was always grateful for anything that helped Keri, even if, on this occasion, the road to get there was a very challenging one!

15

Planning

Planning Permission for Keri's house became our next battle. We were refused Planning Permission 3 times on various sites over this journey. I never saw that battle coming! Early in the process, to my astonishment, I was asked to bring Keri into the planning office to prove that she was as disabled as the medical reports had described. To this day, I cannot fathom how this was seen as an acceptable demand to make of any family and child in our circumstances. The process of getting Planning Permission and the blocks put in our way reminded me so much of the battle with the HSE over the years; there were problems and obstacles at every turn.

Mark and Stephen worked very hard on our campaign to build the right house for Keri. Copious medical reports were required to prove Keri's disability, but queries and clarifications continued to be returned to us from the planners.

Eventually, our planning battle came to a truce, also with the extra help of a local counsellor, Jimmy O'Brien, but not without expensive, awkward and cumbersome conditions laid down by the planners. Finally, we were allowed to 'turn sod' on our new home in Garrinch. This was an enormous milestone for us.

Negotiating an appropriate building contract for Keri's home was time consuming. As the Office of the Wards of Court were (correctly) so careful with Keri's fund, three building tenders were required to be submitted to the Court for consideration. All three contractors are required to have proven experience in building homes for clients with special needs. One of my pre-requisites was that the house be completed in six months, as it had, by then, become almost impossible to care for Keri in our former home. Eventually, MMD Construction was selected, which I was pleased with, as they guaranteed to complete the build within 6 months.

The home for Keri was designed with her in mind at every turn. There was to be no space or corner throughout that Keri couldn't access. This made for a far bigger floor area, but I was adamant that Keri should be able to go to any part of her home at any stage without hindrance. She was never going to be excluded from anything because of her disability, and if that meant a larger home footprint, so be in.

I did not have time to shop around for materials-slabs, slates, flooring, etc., so I was grateful that Mark and Stephen brought me samples to each of our weekly meetings, and I was able to direct things in this fashion.

I had 100% confidence in the team and considered us so blessed. I made it very clear to everyone the importance of this build and that there was no space whatsoever for error. The team delivered. Six months after the ground was broken, we were ready to wheel Keri into her well-appointed, comfortable, peaceful new home.

The new house was built specifically with Keri's funds, especially for Keri. We made every effort to ensure it was her nest, not anything like a hospital, but a safe place to relax and grow, as she and her sister Lucy so truly deserved. Fr Breen visited the week we moved in, and he blessed our home, making it extra special. Keri had her own spacious bedroom, interlinked with the master bedroom for ease of access during the night as she woke countless times during the night if she slept at all. Also interlinked with her bedroom was her wet room, which was a complete luxury. I could now shower Keri with complete confidence that she was safe, secure, and warm. It consisted of a wheelchair accessible shower, a large changing bench and a hoist in between to ensure safe access to and from the shower. She had a hydrotherapy pool, a room for her therapies and equipment, and adequate space for her to chill out in her large open plan kitchen/living area. In a large floor area, special equipment doesn't take over. The room can absorb it, making it less of a 'facility' and more of a home.

Outside our front door, we constructed a large overhang to protect Keri from the wind and rain as she went into and off her bus. Any gust of wind would catch Keri's breath and oftentimes cause a seizure. Furthermore, the wind frequently instigated eye infections. Keri required protection from the rain. The overhang was one of the most important and helpful features of Keri's house, liberating her to get out and about in her bus without the volatility of the Irish weather causing her any further difficulties.

16

Separation

The new house for Keri came together, but my marriage had fallen apart. While the difficulties were apparent when I was pregnant with Lucy, I had remained hopeful that something might change after Lucy was born, but this was not to be. I knew our marriage was well and truly over. There was nothing between us anymore. I was desperately lonely, and I felt we were living a lie.

Chalkie and I lived in the same home, but we lived completely separate lives. I was not the same carefree person Chalkie had married-so much had happened, and so much had changed. In my previous life, my focus was on fun, going out enjoying the nightlife, when life was pretty much carefree, but once Keri came into my life, she was my priority, before anyone or anything else, as was Lucy, when she subsequently arrived.

While Chalkie loved Keri, he really struggled with what had happened to her at birth. He could not find forgiveness, and I totally understood that, but my focus was on Keri, not the past-I didn't have space for both. In some ways, I had to become quite hardened and stubborn in my resolve to see to Keri's welfare. I had to do things for Keri that no parent should have to do, but it wasn't about me, it was always about her. There was no time for backward glances, and there was too much to be done. From my perspective, it was a case of asking Chalkie to step up to the bar or leave me to it. Once we discussed and acknowledged that our marriage was long since over, the reality of separation kicked in, and the psychological dark cloud over me started to lift. We were to split up, having agreed that I alone would move into the new house with Keri and Lucy. Chalkie would remain living in our former home. It was the start of yet another new chapter for us.

Separating was one of the toughest events in my life to date. It was difficult for the Sweeney and Brett families, too. Gossip and rumours infiltrated the town. People astounded me with their ability to feed off our misery and invent stories as to what had happened between us and why. I found this extremely hurtful. I had nothing to hide, and I had done nothing wrong. Neither of us was unfaithful to the other. Life had simply got difficult, and we had, bit by bit, drifted apart. Having our two incredible children together was not sufficient reason to stay together; we were both just too unhappy. We legally separated on the 25th of July, 2013. There was nothing easy about it, but it was the right thing to do. We have two wonderful children together, we remained friends, and by separating, we gave them a happier life, which was all that mattered in the end.

There were endings and beginnings for us all with the move to Garrinch. Keri and Lucy were now children of separated parents, but they no longer lived in an unhappy home. Chalkie conceded that he wouldn't be in a position to look after Keri on a full-time basis, so it was agreed that the girls would live with me, and Chalkie would care for them each week during agreed times/dates. Lucy was four years old, so two big changes at once certainly took some adjusting. Keri was immediately happier with the move. For all of us, having a home specially built for Keri's needs was like stepping into a light at the end of a very dark tunnel.

Stepping into the house in Garrinch is like stepping into the light. As you enter the main door, an expansive hallway greets you, with large glazing pulling the eye directly to the back garden. Neutral colour tones, bright, clean floor tiles and wide corridors make for a welcoming, bright, positive space that lifts the spirits. To allow Keri's wheelchair to glide from room to room, we omitted saddle boards on the floor between rooms, opting instead for a smooth, continuous, clean flooring, which works a treat to seamlessly connect rooms.

I will always remember my very first evening in the new house, showering Keri in her large wheelchair accessible shower. With the changing bench at one side, the shower trolley at the other and a hoist in between, for the first time in her life, Keri and I were fully equipped for a safe, dignified, comfortable shower. Later that evening, when the girls were asleep in bed, I changed into my pyjamas, sat down with the monitor beside me on the corner of the sofa and crunched a bowl of dry Special K to my heart's content while watching television. This was my own piece of heaven, and I could not believe all that we had achieved. It was more than I could have dreamed of for Keri and Lucy. Keri now had everything she needed.

Keri's hydrotherapy pool granted her pure and utter luxury in which to relax and do her stretches with warmth, comfort and ease. It was fantastic for muscle relaxation, which she so deserved after all she was going through. Needless to say, Lucy loved it, too!

The house was designed to be easily kept clean so as to protect Keri's health. We installed a heat recovery air filtration system in the house, which not only regulates ambient temperature in the home but also distributes clean, filtered air throughout the house at all times. Once Keri moved to Garrinch, she suffered far less chest infections, as there was no stagnated unclean air in her environment. Our new home was also far easier to navigate with a wheelchair and equipment on a clean, hard floor rather than a carpet.

An added benefit to the tiled floors was that Keri, with her incredibly sharp hearing, would differentiate who was around her by the sound of their footsteps. She could hear me, a mile off, coming with my heels. I love my high heels, but I also wore them constantly as a way for Keri to know that Mammy was nearby. Cora, who was known to us for her wearing of flip flops, she would be heard with her flip flops down the hall, as I would say, 'Here comes flippy floppy Cora,' causing Keri's face to light up. Keri was very much in touch with her surroundings in her new home, using her various senses to the best of her ability. Her facial expressions told us everything.

When it comes to my children, I am a sucker for meaningful, sentimental items. Instead of decorating our new hall with a painting we purchased, I decided we should make our very own. I acquired a large roll of canvas and laid it out on the hall floor. Over a fortnight, we decorated it. We put paint on the wheels of Keri's chair and rolled her up and down the canvas so she would have her imprint on it. We painted Lucy's feet, and she walked up and down the canvas. Both Keri and Lucy added their hand prints a number of times as the years went by, dating them each time. Carrie, Kate, Jack and Emily Davey all painted whatever they wished, as did whoever wished to leave an imprint. Cora painted her flip flops and signed 'flippy Cora'. It was great fun. When it was complete, Trevor from Melbourne Glass in Clonmel visited to stretch the canvas to a frame he had prepared. He did a wonderful job, and the picture is still perfectly mounted today. As the years went by, we added to the canvas. It is such a beautiful reminder of our happy memories throughout the years. It is an artwork we created together, one of a kind.

From day one, Lucy slept with Keri in her bedroom, a very special routine for the girls. Her room was personalised, like for any other little girls, with a floor to ceiling display of games, books and teddies. I dressed the girls' beds in dusky pink bed linen, soft and welcoming for their precious little bodies. Keri's bed was a specialised four-foot hospital bed, which was quite high. Lucy's was a standard, which was lower.

It was suggested to me by OT Joanne that I purchase Lucy a second mattress so that she could be elevated and level beside Keri to hold her hand to bring Lucy comfort. My two girls slept hand in hand, Lucy cuddling into Keri every night. They were two peas in a pod. Lucy told me she felt safe with Keri, even though she knew Keri couldn't do anything if there was a problem. Lucy's bedroom became her playroom. Her place of rest was with her precious big sister.

For the rest of Keri's life, my two girls slept together. It was so special to see on the monitor two devoted sisters taking such good care of each other. Keri never slept through the night, but she did her very best. The girls slept with a very dimly lit lamp in the bedroom, as Keri was terrified of the dark. Not only was the light reassuring for Keri, but it also illuminated the scene for me for the essential overnight nappy changes. Over time, I became adept at making these changes without disturbing Keri. A good night would have been four or five awakenings where I would come in to settle Keri, a bad night may see Keri never settling at all. Thankfully, however, Lucy always slept through.

I remember watching a television programme titled 'DIY SOS', and the building was for a child with a similar disability to Keri. I found it so emotional to watch, as I suddenly realised that I had provided Keri with the same luxury-I realised the enormity of it. I felt so proud of myself. Money could never buy Keri's health, but I had been able to achieve so much to make her life easier.

The girls settled in quickly to their new life at home in Garrinch. I saw a huge change in them. Keri had every luxury she could wish for, and she was certainly much more relaxed. Lucy was so excited by the newness of everything. She loved feeding apples to the neighbouring horses, a daily ritual she established soon after we moved in. I purchased her a small scooter to use inside the house, and she absolutely loved it, whizzing up and down the hall, delighted with herself. The girls brought such a happy, positive energy to the home. I dotted photographs in every corner of the house to celebrate all our happy times together. The children adored the company of wild rabbits, deer and foxes in our gorgeous rural garden. We were blessed with really wonderful, welcoming, and helpful neighbours, which was a huge comfort to me. We developed a lovely relationship with them all.

It had taken from late 2009 to September 2011 to get to this point, but it was worth the wait and hard work. In her new space, our little butterfly could spread her wings and blossom into her best self. The new home for Keri was undoubtedly the biggest tangible benefit from the court case. This home was to be Keri's safe place for the rest of her days.

17

Mass

Safe and happy in our new home, the daily routine continued. I rolled on with Keri's Physiotherapy programme to help her with various physical symptoms and avoid further curvature of the spine, which was starting to cause her distress. While the Zanaflex was really helping Keri relax, the feeding was becoming quite problematic-the curvature was obscuring her positioning for feeding, which resulted in significant weight loss. Dr Condon and the CRC in Waterford did everything they could to prevent further curvature, as did I, with as much Physiotherapy at home as we could manage, overseen by Raj, her physiotherapist, and Joanne and Dan, her local Occupational therapists.

Once we were settled into the new house, I began taking my two girls to Mass, usually on Sundays. I felt it was important to teach the girls the customs and traditions of a Roman Catholic Mass, as their holy sacraments of communion and confirmation were coming up. In our local church, we found our own little cosy spot to sit, where we could be found each week. This was where Fr Breen, our then parish priest and long-time family friend, would visit us. He always made a habit of speaking with us and making a fuss of Keri before each and every service. One particular Sunday, Fr Breen was late, so he got himself robed up and went straight to the altar to start the service. Keri was not a bit happy. This was not the normal routine, as she didn't get her usual greeting. She shouted the church down throughout the entire Mass! Even when I took her out of her chair for a cuddle, she would not stop. It was so funny; Fr Breen had her spoiled. After mass, he came down to say hello, and he was greeted with the biggest, most beautiful smile ever. Keri was now happy.

Mass was a huge event in our week. It was a social outing for us, and we got to know more about the local community. People would speak with Keri and us all after the service, and we all got to know each other as parishioners. It meant so much to us; mass was a great blessing in so many ways and gave us all a huge sense of comfort and belonging.

Keri was very well able to take her rightful place in the world. When certain close family and friends would come in the door of our home, Keri's eyes would light up with a dazzling smile. Not everyone got this welcome. For some, her head would go down, and she wouldn't acknowledge them. Equally, if a person met Keri and only spoke to me, Keri (rightly) would raise a huge objection. She would leave out one hell of a shout, where I would have to explain that one must say hello to Keri and include her in the conversation. She must not be ignored or left out. Over time, thankfully, this became the norm, such that Keri would be greeted before I was, which suited me just fine.

Keri had a special relationship with her hairdresser, Stephanie, who always had the biggest welcome for her in her salon. Keri was awarded the freedom of Stephanie's salon, which she adored! She got free haircuts anytime she needed one as she sat up in my lap as proud as punch.

Keri had her own circle of friends, people I didn't even know. Oftentimes, as we strolled and wheeled through the town, people would say hello to her, people that I didn't even recognise. She brought the best out in everyone. No matter how bad a day people were having, once they saw Keri, they always smiled. She was like a lightning bolt. She had the most special, energising and healing energy that people were drawn to.

Around this time, Keri's eyesight was becoming more problematic. Up to that point, Keri had been attending Waterford Regional Hospital and the CRC for eye tests. While it was an excellent service, the prolonged waiting periods before she would be seen became less feasible. Due to the increased curvature in her spine, Keri was showing increasing discomfort in sitting for a prolonged period; she would only tolerate the chair for a short period before she would be required to lie out. She was no longer able to handle the long wait times for appointments.

I managed to secure a private appointment with an ophthalmologist, which became our new system. The staff were so accommodating, and they even posted eye drops to me in advance of appointments, which saved us time on arrival. Those little gestures make a huge difference to families like ours. We worked with Conor Fleming, a local optician in Clonmel who provided an excellent and personalised service. Conor and Keri got on great, and Keri really enjoyed her visits.

Conor always included Keri in the discussions about her eyes. The assistants were always so welcoming to Keri, and it became a place we looked forward to visiting. Getting the right frame for Keri was never a difficulty. The staff worked hard to ensure that she got a nice colourful frame, especially featuring her well known favourites, pink or purple. With Keri's scoliosis, she tended to lean to one side, so Conor calibrated the frames to remain level on her little face.

As time moved on, Keri became more light sensitive. Moving from the indoors to the outdoors oftentimes provoked seizure activity. Keri also suffered a number of eye infections. Sometimes, even the wind would cause an infection. Eventually, I noticed that when Keri wore sunglasses, she was less sensitive, so Conor suggested we try transition lenses, which worked a treat for Keri. As she transitioned to and from different light shades, her lenses would slowly transition to accommodate the light so she wouldn't get a fright. Conor and his team examined options from all angles to ensure Keri's glasses were as clear, comfortable and, above all, stylish for our beautiful princess.

The Court case was well and truly behind us, funds were available for a care package, but I had no intention of stepping down as Keri's primary carer. I wanted to do it myself, as much as possible. However, I knew that if I kept going as I was, I would run myself into the ground. While Chalkie always took the girls out on a Sunday afternoon, there otherwise wasn't a formal arrangement in place; it would very much depend on Chalkie's availability and Keri's form.

Getting very little sleep was taking its toll, and between trying to keep the house in order, look after the girls and attend appointments, I was finding it hard. I knew I had to put some more help in place to ease the pressure. If I wasn't right, I couldn't give the girls 100%. As I always say, you need to fill your cup in order to give to others.

At that time, Cora was working Saturdays from 10am to 5pm, but she also helped me on other occasions by request if she could. My mother suggested I get some assistance with the housework, and my sister Fionnuala agreed to help. She started coming over on Tuesday and Friday mornings. Fionnuala, a mother of four herself, was somebody I could trust implicitly in our home, and she always cleaned the house to perfection. She was very happy to help with Keri if I needed it.

While Keri was tricky to look after, and lots of people were frightened of her condition, Fionnuala had no difficulty. When she was in the house, if I needed to pop into Fethard, I could leave Keri with Fionnuala. In terms of travel, especially when ill, vomiting was a big problem for Keri and a concern for me, as there was a risk of aspiration, which could lead to pneumonia. If there was an appointment to be attended and if Keri was unwell, Fionnuala would oblige if possible. It was always a great support and peace of mind to have someone in the back of the bus with Keri while I drove when Keri needed extra support, as we had to be so careful with her chest. All of Keri's carers throughout the years were great in that regard, too.

18

Romance

Marita has been one of my best friends for over twenty-five years at this stage. A pharmacy assistant with the a big heart, we met socialising in Fethard enjoying a laugh over many drinks, beating the roads together, trying to keep the weight down. She and her husband Brian lived in Strylea, across the road from us, in our previous family home, where they remain to date. Marita is full of life, great company and incredible crack to be around. She has enhanced my life with fun, laughter and madness, and indeed, she continues to.

It was the 20th of April 2012, and we were living in the new house for a month. Marita and I had planned a night out in Clonmel together, as we occasionally would when Keri's health allowed. At that time, after a separation and house move, not to mention ongoing worries about Keri, my frame of mind was just to go out with Mairita, have a good laugh, drink and dance the legs off ourselves, releasing from the pressures of life. When Marita and I go out, it is just us in our bubble of fun. We don't engage with the rest of the world. We just have a good few drinks, lots of laughs together and dance to our heart's content. That night, we went to a few pubs for a few drinks and then went to O'Keeffe's disco bar. As we were out on the dance floor, I could see this bloke on the higher end-where there was another bar, looking down, smiling at me on the dance floor. I caught him looking at me a few times and said to myself, 'What is that ape smiling at? If only he knew of my baggage!' I also genuinely believed that nobody would ever fancy me, so I didn't take any more notice. I just thought he was being nice.

We left the floor and returned to our drinks. The 'smiling chap' approached us. He asked me how I was and if I was having a good night. I just couldn't believe he was trying to chat me up. I was totally taken aback. He told me his name was Mark. I told him to go away and that he must be full of drink. He said he was not, that he was only on his third pint. Mark said he wasn't even planning to go out, but his friend asked him to come out for a drink at the last minute, and he obliged. I told him that I am complicated. He asked what I meant by this, and I asked him to go away, saying that I had no interest in romance, that I was recently out of a marriage and only one month out of the home, and that I have two children, one of whom is severely disabled. His answer to me was, 'Well, so what, sure, isn't she still a child?' This response sparked an interest in me. Not every man would respond in such a fashion. Mark asked if we could exchange numbers and arrange to meet for a coffee. I agreed. We exchanged numbers, and that was it. Later that night, the Budweiser caught up on me, and although I do not remember it, I rang him in the middle of the night. He didn't have a clue what I was saying, and by the sounds of it, nor did I!

Mark sent me a text message the following week and asked that we meet for coffee. I agreed. Mark was living in Clonmel at the time. We met in BB's at the showgrounds. We met during school hours, as I was free during this period, and he was working nights at the time. He told me that he was also separated and had two daughters. We remarked that there wasn't much of an age gap between his youngest girl and Keri. I told him about my girls. He was really interested in Keri and her additional needs. He wanted to know their ages, their interests and their personalities. I explained that everything was still so complicated in my life after the recent separation and that although we had lived separate lives for quite some time-that I wasn't after a relationship; nor on the lookout that night!

His answer was that perhaps it was the right time and the right place. Mark was separated for a number of years by then and was interested in meeting someone. I made it perfectly clear from this first coffee together that the girls were and always would be my absolute priority.

Mark and I met a few times from then on for a coffee, but the girls were never around. I was so surprised at how naturally the conversations flowed and how comfortable

I felt around him. Mark was so pleasant to talk to, and he expected nothing from me. There was no agenda. We clicked straight away. We enjoyed friendly, free flowing, adult conversations. Within three weeks, we knew we had something worth continuing. We knew we had feelings for each other. When you know, you know.

A month later, I introduced Mark to Keri and Lucy. Mark called out to our house, and he was immediately a natural with them. He was really taken aback by my two girls. Given Keri had so many needs, he was intrigued by her fun-loving personality and various preferences, particularly for colour, music and style. Lucy was initially shy and in my arms-she was very small at the time, but after 15 minutes, she started to loosen up and play with Mark, jumping up on his belly, which Lucy thought was hilarious. It was a child-centred get-together, and I was just thrilled it had gone so well. I just couldn't believe I had met someone so generous and warm-hearted that I got another chance at happiness. From the very beginning, Mark was a great support. He treated Keri as a child first, with a disability second, rather than the other way around. It was so refreshing and such a joy to witness.

After Mark's meeting with the girls, I told Chalkie I had met someone. I said we wanted to give it a go and see how it went. Chalkie seemed unaffected by the news. I arranged to see his mother, and I told her. She didn't take it so well. The news was upsetting for her, which I understood. A lot of people in the town had their opinions, and the rumour mill restarted, but I had nothing to be ashamed of. I had done no wrong. I couldn't apologise for falling in love, and I knew I deserved to be happy.

As time moved along, Mark and I continued to see each other. On a Sunday, Chalkie would take the girls for their usual time together and Mark and I would go for a coffee. It was all so simple and relaxed. Once we knew that we really wanted things to progress, Mark introduced me to his daughter, Kym, and his other daughter, Kelly, who lived in Jersey with her mum. He brought Kym out to our house. She was 6 years old at the time. Keri, Lucy and I were all there to meet her, and it went really well. Kym played with Lucy and was comfortable around us all. Mark and I were thrilled. It was delightful that the girls got on so well. We knew it was only baby steps, and we were happy to proceed in that fashion. On a Saturday, Kym used to horse ride so Mark would spend the day with her. We were by no means living in each other's pockets. My girls were my priority, and Kym was his. We didn't do any more for a long time than just meet up for a coffee. We took it slowly.

On the 1st of June, 2012, we celebrated Keri's First Holy Communion, which took place in Rosegreen Church. It was a beautiful, intimate service, as there were only a few children in Keri's school group who were of age to go forward for the sacrament. After the service, we enjoyed exquisite refreshments at the hall in Rosegreen Church with all the teachers and carers. Then we returned home and enjoyed my brother Liam's catering with family and friends. My dear friend Sharon had travelled from the UK specially to join Keri for her special day. Keri's proud and devoted Godfather, Buda, wouldn't have missed the occasion for all the world; always such a great support to us. Mark came round later that evening when most of the crowd had departed. This was the occasion of Mark's first meeting with my family.

When my family met Mark, some didn't make it easy for him. Everybody was so protective of me, after all I had been through and because of the ill-founded notion out there that I had money from Keri's court case. My family saw me as vulnerable.

The truth is that Keri had money from her Court case, and that money was lodged in Court, paid out on application to the President of the High Court for her welfare. I was paid a modest rate (but perfectly acceptable to me) by the Court to care for her. I lived in Keri's house; it was not mine. The first Mark knew there was 'money' there was when one of my family asked him straight out if he was there for the right reasons. They were concerned that he was attracted to the large house, which might suggest I was a rich lady. Mark said he didn't know anything about 'money' and that he was there to be with me. Mark had to work hard to get my family's approval. It took time to build trust. When we were in London, in Great Ormond Street Children's Hospital, Mammy said to Mark that she could see he was with us for the right reasons. He was there to do everything he could to help. She saw he was an utterly genuine man. We finally had her blessing. As Mammny was and still is such a massive part of my life, this meant the world to me.

Lucy was growing up fast. She attended a local dance school, 'On Your Toes Academy,' and every year, they rolled out an end of year performance, which we all very proudly attended. It was normally held over two nights, so we would share the nights between us so that somebody would always be in attendance for Lucy. Mary, Chris, Cathal, Amanda, Fionnuala and her son Mark, Chalkie, Mark, Keri and I all enjoyed the shows so much. Madge, the principal of the academy, always made sure we had front row seats to allow us to bring Keri. Keri loved being in the middle of things and was so proud to see her little sister on stage, with the added bonus of meeting lots of new friendly faces. We always looked forward to and enjoyed these nights out, and we were so proud of Lucy. She was growing into the finest young lady imaginable.

19

Curvature

I had been truly blessed to have Mark come into our lives. He brought us such joy, comfort and contentment. He had a wonderful way with the girls. When we talk about the night we met, Mark would say to me that he saw a woman who just stood out so much on the dance floor that I seemed to really enjoy myself, maybe a bit of a lunatic in the nicest way, that I was really letting my hair down. He was attracted by the fun coming from our corner. Mark told me some time later that when he saw me on the dance floor, he turned to his friend Owen and announced, 'I am going to marry her'. I always thought that was a joke, but I later learned this was true. He had indeed said that to Owen.

Mark and I work together as a team. We can rely on each other and speak openly about anything. If something is upsetting Mark, he can talk about it. He will cry in front of me; he is no big tough man but is in touch with his feminine side. We always put an effort into our time as a couple. We try to spend time together, to make space for one another and our togetherness, even if only for a coffee and a chat.

I had no doubt that Keri and Lucy adored Mark. Keri's eyes would beam up at him. She would smile so broadly as he would play with her, and she loved her cuddles with him. He would make an eejit of himself just to make her smile, no matter who was in the room. Mark would do anything just to distract Keri from pain, just to ease her suffering and make her laugh. He always maintained, just like the first night we met, that she was a child first. Lucy took to Mark really well. She loved the attention from him, their playing and fooling about. When we had a family day out, she loved having Mark there, too. Lucy was always so mindful that she also had her Dad, Chalkie, and carefully ensured he knew that he was important to her, too. She would never have wanted to hurt him. Once Mark came into my life, we all became winners.

The timing of this blossoming relationship turned out to be ideal, as things were getting particularly difficult. While we had a wonderful celebration for Keri's First Holy Communion, she was, at that time, becoming extremely thin and gaunt. Arising from her spinal curvature, she was experiencing a lot of discomfort when eating and drinking, which was, as time went on, cumulatively taking up to 8 hours a day. Her school attendance was falling off, as she was frequently unable to do it, and her bouts of crying and distress noticeably increased. The Botox injections were no longer providing Keri with the relief they once did. Her condition had become more complex, and her suffering far more pronounced.

I was becoming overwhelmed. I was struggling with years of compounded exhaustion, and I needed more help. Luckily, I was introduced to an outstanding lady by the name of Ruth Higgins, Marita's sister-in-law, a qualified, trained, experienced special needs carer. She was available for a few hours two days a week, and her input became both a source of joy for the girls and a help to me. Ruth was an absolute dream with Keri, and if Lucy was at home, Ruth always ensured to include her in everything. I was exhausted from the hydrotherapy pool, but it was really beneficial for Keri, so I had to do it daily, no matter how I was feeling. Once Ruth came on board, she was very happy to do it on her two days, which was a huge relief to me, and it made a pleasant change for Keri.

Cora continued to work with us on a Saturday morning, which was fantastic. When Cora or Ruth worked with Keri, I was in a position to do the grocery shopping, go to the gym for an hour or take a walk, breaks I truly needed. Cora and Ruth were a godsend during this time. The Sweeney and Brett families, together with Chalkie, also helped in any way they could. I needed all the support I could get. Things were, physically and mentally, exceptionally difficult.

Lucy was feeling it, too. There was no protecting her from the reality of her sister's extraordinary suffering. Oftentimes, when Keri was in distress, Lucy, who was only six years of age at the time, would sit up beside her ten year old big sister and say, 'I wish I could make you all better'. She just wanted to be with Keri, make her smile and comfort her. In all the relentless crying and distress, day and night, over weeks and weeks, Lucy would sometimes look over to me and ask, 'Will Keri die?' My heart would break. All I could do was love and try to comfort these two remarkable little angels, but I could not deny the reality of Keri's condition. She was getting much, much more unwell.

By November 2013, Keri was eleven years old and enduring ongoing enormous pain and discomfort. The curvature of her spine had drastically deteriorated, her little trunk had twisted, and the lower right side of her ribcage was now meeting the front bone of her pelvis. The ribcage and pelvis would painfully rub together with every move and transfer. Her ribcage was sharply protruding with significant pressure, such that, as time went on, I became terrified that the lower part of her ribcage would break through her skin; she was so thin that her bones were barely covered.

This dreadful curvature was severely impacting all of Keri's internal organs, particularly her digestive system. Her food would become jammed in the abdomen, with nowhere to go, causing her enormous pain, particularly late in the evening. Keri was losing her hard earned weight. Feeding was really hurting her. The calories she was using to feed were far more than I was able to get into her. During this time, the crying was relentless, and I walked the floors of our home through the night every night with Keri in my arms.

Although Keri was small, this was especially physically and emotionally draining for me. There was no settling Keri, no medication that would ease her pain. Her twisted body shape was now torturing her. I was devastated that we had now arrived at this point; I knew it was a further deterioration in her overall condition. I also wished to see Keri enjoy her food for as long as possible, but this pleasure had long since passed, surpassed by the pain and distress that the feeding was causing her. As hard as it was to accept, I took the advice from the CRC that a PEG feeding tube was the kindest solution for Keri. A referral was made to the children's hospital.

Keri was in dire straits, but this was of no concern to the HSE. She was not their priority. Keri was merely placed on a lifeless hospital waiting list, while every second of her every day inflicted further vicious pain and suffering upon her. My appeals to the hospital to admit her fell on deaf ears. I contacted politicians and families of politicians, who did all they could for Keri, but to no avail. We waited and waited while Keri became more and more tortured.

Meanwhile, it was recommended that Keri see a neurologist to investigate her deteriorating condition. We were placed at the end of another enormous HSE waiting list for a consultation. Once again, I took matters into my own hands. I arranged a private appointment with Dr Niamh Lynch, a Paediatric Neurologist at the Bon Secours Hospital in Cork. Dr Lynch admitted Keri to the hospital to get a complete workup done and consider the various options. It was a huge relief to have Dr Lynch take control of the situation. Between the unknown of what was to come, not being able to help Keri feel better, the worry of her deterioration and the upset this was causing Lucy, I was almost at breaking point. I was feeling helpless, overwhelmed, and exhausted.

Dr Lynch arranged for Keri to have an EEG (Electroencephalogram) to investigate seizure activity by detecting abnormalities in Keri's brainwave pattern. I requested that an MRI also be carried out to see the extent of Keri's spinal curvature and the adverse effect this was having on her internal organs. I had been calling for this investigation for some time from the HSE, but to no avail. I was delighted that Dr Lynch agreed to it. I believe Keri must have known of the importance of this scan, as she stayed utterly still throughout, so much so that they did not even have to sedate her. Keri was so exhausted from her endless crying that she slept throughout despite the almost deafening noise from the machine. I was allowed to stay with Keri every step of the way.

The staff were incredibly skilled and supportive. I was fed lovely meals all throughout our stay. Every doctor considered a possible help to Keri was called upon for a consultation. Every conceivable test was carried out to identify all sources of her pain and discomfort. Her well-being was at the forefront of minds at the Bons. A pressure relief air mattress was ordered for Keri, with the hope that it would give her gaunt little body some relief. Unfortunately, it did not suit Keri- as the movement frightened her, it caused even further distress, but it was no difficulty for the staff to simply replace it. Trial and error is the only way we can learn what suits children like Keri. Sadly, there is no other formula.

Luckily, Mark moved in for a period during this time to help look after Lucy. Chalkie helped out, too. Chalkie's brother Cathal, Lucy's Godfather and his partner Amanda have been a massive support to us ever since Keri was born. When Mark worked nights, Cathal and Amanda took Lucy and her friend Aine for sleepovers, keeping her well entertained and distracted. 'Aunty Amanda' is a qualified childminder, and my girls always enjoyed her various tricks to entertain them. Lucy's friends and their families-Perry, Mandy, Ed, Lorraine, Noelle, PJ, Liam and Teresa, were a further enormous source of help, taking Lucy for sleepovers and fun days out. These people kept our family going.

During Keri's time in Cork, the hospital where Keri so urgently needed to go was contacted daily by the team to enquire about bed availability for her. Day after day, such endeavours proved fruitless. Once again, politicians were petitioned to see if they could assist. The staff in the Bon Secours were amazed how I had not 'cracked up' with the pressure and heartbreak during this time. Keri was suffering so much, and the crying was unrelenting. I kept the fire in my belly ignited to fight for Keri at every turn. All the while, with my best game face on, I had no other choice. It did, of course, break my heart to witness such suffering of my little angel; she would look up at me with her big green eyes begging for my help, but I simply could not let it overwhelm me. I didn't carry anger or resentment for the circumstances surrounding Keri's birth, but the neglect by the HSE in caring for her at excruciating times such as this, when she was suffering such relentless, agonising pain, enraged me like never before. I battled as hard as I ever had. I didn't care how much I annoyed people, Keri was all that mattered. Every day that I was ignored, I got twice as angry and fought twice as hard the next day. This circus of pestering, declines and disappointment went on and on and on. All the while, Keri screamed and writhed in ever increasing agony while her little sister was without her Mum and big sister for weeks on end. Some days did get the better of me, and I cried with pure distraught trying to fathom out how the system was such a letdown to my beautiful, innocent Keri, and I could not take away her pain.

Yet another Friday arrived, the end of another long week with no bed in sight for Keri. She had now been in Cork for three weeks, and we were both yearning to get home to Lucy. The hospital agreed to discharge Keri for the weekend so we could have some family time, upon the understanding that we could return at any stage if Keri deteriorated. I was in a position to administer all her medication, and I felt she might as well scream the house down as scream the hospital down. At least we would be at home as a family. I promptly packed up our belongings and set off on the road home. Lucy wasn't expecting me to collect her from school that afternoon, so it was an extremely special surprise reunion for us both. 'Mammyyyyyyyyy', she cried, as her little surprised face spotted me at the school gates. She ran to me, jumped into my arms, and we clung to each other for the longest time in our gorgeous reunion. It was like something you would see in a movie. I can still feel those butterflies in my belly today when I think of that moment; I had missed Lucy so much over those weeks in Cork. It was heart wrenching to be away from her for so long.

That weekend was difficult as Keri was so unwell and so upset, but we made the most of our time together. I knew we would be on the road to Cork again on Sunday evening for a further painfully undefined period of separation. It was so difficult to hold things together. Mark made a world of difference in supporting me and the girls; he really was such a blessing to us all. Knowing Lucy was with Cathal and Amanda also gave me great comfort with the help of her dad too, where possible

Sunday evening arrived too fast. We said our goodbyes before Keri and I headed off for Cork once again. I got back to work on the telephone on Monday to ascertain if there were any positive developments on a bed for Keri, to which I got the same bad news. Keri continued to scream in distress, and there was nothing that could be done for her but to sit and wait in the hope a bed would become available. Its beggared belief that a first world country like Ireland would treat its most vulnerable, sick children like this. Eventually, after countless further phone calls and pressure, a bed was offered to Keri in the hospital at the end of that week. I was gobsmacked that it required the lobbying and pressure of a politician to get Keri the basic help she most urgently required. If a dog was in a similar predicament of pain and distress, it would have the help offered sooner than to a child. I saw and continue to see it as an absolute shame and disgrace to our society.

Keri was offered a transfer by ambulance, but I elected to transfer her myself. Keri's bus was parked just outside the hospital door, and I knew if she was given sufficient medication to make her comfortable for the three-hour journey, we would manage just as well. We set off collecting Mammy on the way. She had her bag packed, ready to join and support us as soon as we were able to travel.

I breathed a sigh of relief as we entered the motorway, firmly believing there was light at the end of the tunnel and that Keri's suffering would soon be behind her. I was exhausted, such was the fight to have her admitted to the designated hospital. Little did I realise I would have to dig well into my reserves once we arrived. Another battle lay ahead for us, having just about crawled, exhausted, and depleted out of the last one. An error had been made in noting Keri's date of birth. The hospital was expecting a baby, not an eleven year old. We were told to go home, that there were no children's beds available. Keri screamed her heart out in reception, and the staff could see for themselves the predicament we were in. I made it clear that I didn't care what operational problems they had, Keri's problems were greater, and I bluntly refused to leave the hospital. Eventually, after hours of waiting as Keri screamed, a bed was found for her.

After two days, I sent Mammy home. Things were just so difficult, and I felt I needed to protect her from witnessing the level of brutal suffering Keri was enduring.

Keri underwent a battery of tests during her first week in hospital. She was seen by a paediatric orthopaedic surgeon who examined her and reviewed her history, including her recent radiology images. From the X-ray, the surgeon concluded that Keri's spinal curvature was so severe that it was profoundly affecting her stomach and internal organs. The curvature was also causing her spine to pinch nerves, causing severe nerve pain. She urgently required surgery to straighten her spine, take the pressure off her organs and release her from the torture she was enduring. I was told that Keri would be required to wait for her place on the list for this surgery and that it was likely to be five months before she would undergo the procedure. I reluctantly agreed to the wait, upon the understanding that it would be done at that stage without question.

A barium swallow test was also carried out. This involves swallowing a solution containing barium sulphate, a metallic compound which can easily be seen on an X-ray. As the solution travelled down the gut, it was tracked by X-ray to see if Keri was aspirating her food and liquid. Regrettably, the results were conclusive: Keri was indeed taking food and liquids into her lungs. I had suspected this was the case, but to have it confirmed was heartbreaking.

The time had come for Keri to be fitted with a PEG device, a flexible feeding tube that would be surgically inserted into her abdomen, allowing nutrition, hydration and medication to be administered to her stomach directly, bypassing the mouth and oesophagus, thereby protecting her airways and allowing her to gain and hopefully maintain body mass. Her days of enjoying her dinners were over. It was a poignant milestone in her deterioration, but I had no option, as always, but to fill up my coffee mug and re-apply the game face.

Keri had been in this particular hospital for a week at this stage, and she was still screaming in pain. I had a lot of work to do for her. I was told by the surgeon that Keri would be sent home and that I would be contacted if and when a bed became available in or around May to insert the PEG (it was then March, so that would be at least two months of further waiting).

I was flabbergasted. Keri had been in Cork for almost four weeks, awaiting a transfer for surgery. The tests had now concluded that she was aspirating, a life-threatening condition which would foreseeably lead to pneumonia if not managed with a PEG and now we were simply being sent home to wait some more. I asked the doctor if I was hearing him correctly. Once he confirmed I was, I became hysterical and simply refused to leave the hospital. I told him that they would need an army to physically remove me from the premises. We were going nowhere. I could not believe things had come to this. All the while, Keri continued to scream. I was so physically, mentally and emotionally exhausted. I missed Lucy so much. My precious little child was dying in pain before me, and we were now being shown the door without any help. I sobbed, begging for help, as the doctor turned on his heels and walked away again. Further, insult was heaped upon the injury of my beautiful Keri by the HSE.

I dug my heels in, and we stayed put. I stayed with Keri day and night, sleeping on a cushioned, thick fold away mat. I just couldn't leave her, we needed each other, and I just felt I couldn't trust the system to give her priority. The nursing staff were amazingly understanding towards us. One week later, Keri underwent surgery to have her PEG tube inserted. On arrival to recovery, her little body appeared to be in shock, and she was cold, wrapped in a foil blanket and heavily sedated. As she awoke, she was extremely upset and required a lot of pain relief to settle her. In the time that followed, we worked hard to adapt Keri's little system to the PEG feeds. I underwent significant training in feeding and hygiene of the peg site and equipment. As Keri's system had difficulty breaking down proteins, it took some time to figure out what feed would suit her whilst also meeting her dietary needs. While it was a distressing time for Keri, we had no choice but to persist and figure out her brand new nutritional puzzle.

All the while, Lucy was getting very anxious, and we were all missing each other so much. It had, by now, been six weeks of separation, and while close friends and family had brought Lucy for visits when possible, she was really suffering, and my heart was breaking. Lucy didn't have another sibling to lean on. I wanted her to know that although she wasn't seeing me, she was as loved and as important as Keri at all times. I felt very much between a rock and a hard place. My two children were in different counties, and both desperately needed me.

Mother's Day was approaching, and Lucy begged me to spend it with her. An incredible Nurse suggested I book a hotel near the hospital and take a night away with Lucy. I couldn't imagine leaving Keri alone, so Chalkie agreed to stay with her for the night. The staff would be there to do all her feeds and medications. I booked Lucy and I into a lovely hotel, a treat Lucy so thoroughly deserved. I couldn't wait to spoil her rotten.

As much as I hated leaving Keri, Lucy needed this one-to-one time. We had a wonderful evening together, shopping and dining out before having a 'pamper night' back in our hotel room with the various cosmetics we had purchased earlier that day together. It did us both the world of good. I have a lifelong happy memory of Lucy wrapped up in a huge white bathrobe in the hotel room, so big it trailed behind her little body, as she beamed at me with her big blue eyes, her stunning big smile and her blond curly hair. She always loved hotel breakfasts, and we enjoyed ours the following morning together, bright and early, before heading back to the reality of the hospital. Chalkie and Lucy departed for Tipperary immediately upon our return to Keri's bedside. My heart shattered seeing Lucy go so fast after such a beautiful night, but I hoped it wouldn't be too long before Keri would settle and we would all be home together again.

It took time, but eventually, Keri began to settle. Discussions began about a discharge home. While Keri was still in a lot of pain and distress, she was too thin to have her spinal operation. She needed to put on weight and build up her strength for it. She was commenced on a BuTrans Transdermal patch 5mg to tide her over in terms of pain management until her spinal operation could take place. For now, the insertion of the PEG, together with an increase in her pain medication, was the best that could be done for her. Cruelly, Keri was only two days at home when she became unsettled and started vomiting. As I had been directed, I brought her back to the hospital for review. She was readmitted, and an X-ray was carried out to ascertain if the PEG had dislodged. Thankfully, it was properly in place, so it was a matter of reviewing her feed with the dietician. After some adjustments to her feed, she settled well and was discharged home once again.

I was never so relieved to be heading home. It had been a gruelling six week marathon. Fionnuala had cleaned our house to perfection. There was nothing like the smell of bleach to know our house was clean and safe for Keri, giving extra protection from infection. Ruth arrived shortly after we arrived home. Lucy burst into the house, having returned from school, fizzing with excitement to have us home. Her reaction to seeing us was electric. It was a beautiful, warm spring day. To my great relief, Ruth was very experienced in caring for PEG fed children, so I was free to take in a little peace and quiet, knowing that Keri was perfectly well looked after. Ruth took Keri outside for some well-earned fresh air, and Lucy hurried out after them. I breathed a sigh of relief that this chapter of anguish was now closed. Keri could now be fed safely; her pain was under control, and there was a plan in place to sort out her spinal curvature. We were now back at home, and my gorgeous girls reunited once again.

Music blaring, I jumped into the shower while I had a chance. I could finally enjoy a moment alone time to gather myself and land while the girls enjoyed being outside with Ruth. I emerged from the shower with a towel around me, only to find Chalkie waiting to speak with me.

Prior to Keri's long hospital stay and PEG insertion, Chalkie would usually take Keri for a couple of afternoons a week to spend time with her. However, he explained that things had changed and that he could no longer do it. He said he found the night he spent with Keri in the hospital extremely difficult, and it was still playing on his mind. He said he could no longer cope with her condition, and he didn't think it was fair for Keri to continue as before. He had come to the end of his time with Keri. I knew by talking to him that, nothing would change his mind.

Although initially I was shocked and cross that he thought it was okay to just walk away, when I reflected upon it, I felt it was probably the kindest decision for Keri. He knew that he couldn't cope with all the deteriorations and changes with Keri. While she was the same incredible little girl, her condition was becoming ever more complex and demanding. Ever since her birth, Chalkie had found it hard to come to terms with her brain injury. Now, with a PEG feeding tube inserted and a massive spinal operation coming down the tracks, he knew it was too much for him. At that moment, he did the kindest and most responsible thing, and he gave up his parental rights legally to Keri. It was a choice he made as he believed it to be for the best.

He knew Keri would be best looked after by Mark and I, and she wouldn't want for a thing. In life, things are never black and white.

Life can get complicated and difficult. When it comes to children, we must all know and acknowledge our limitations. I respect his decision and take my hat off to him for doing the right thing for Keri. He knew the girls were my world, and by doing this, I now could get on with caring for Keri myself. It didn't mean that he didn't care for her. He cared for her enough to give her up.

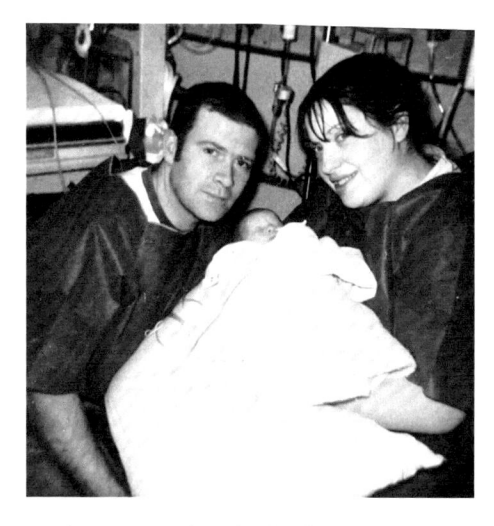

Photo 1 - 21st October 2003, 1 day after her birth with Mum and Dad

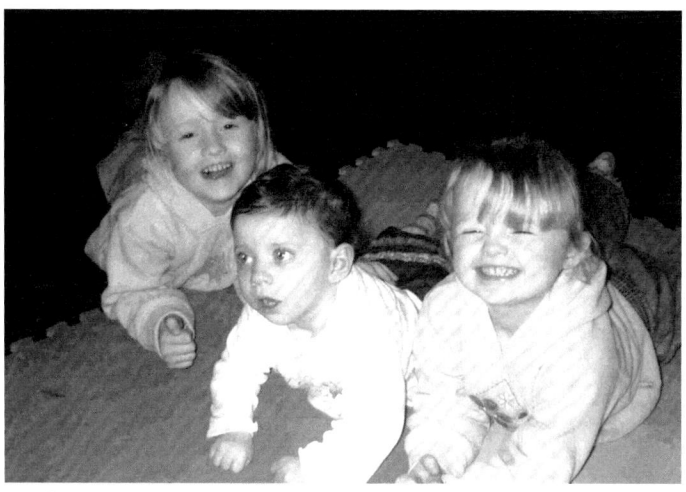

Photo 2 - Kate and Carrie her little therapists after finishing physio

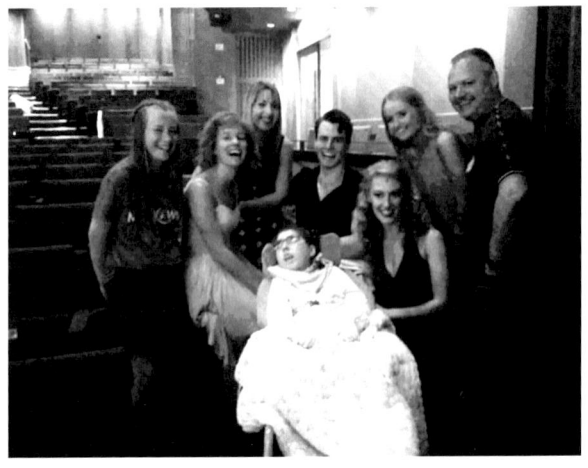

Photo 3 - Meeting some of the cast of Dirty Dancing

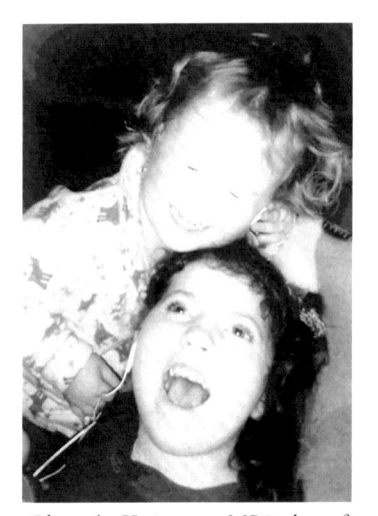

Photo 4 - Keri got an MP3 player from Santa, Lucy was so excited for Keri

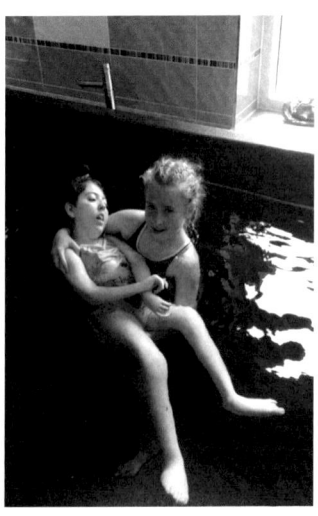

Photo 5 - Keri enjoying her therapy pool

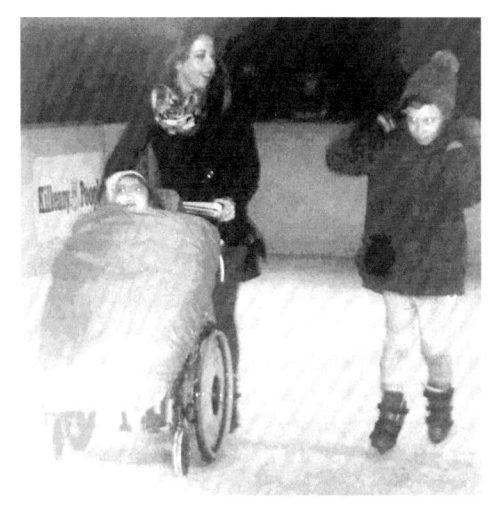

Photo 6 - Keri enjoying Ice skating with her cousin Mark

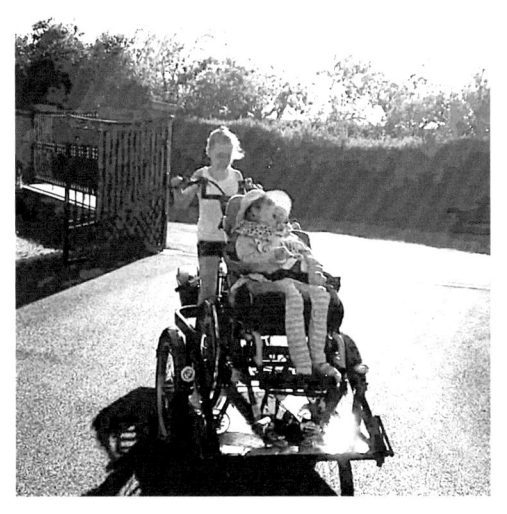

Photo 7 - Keri loving being cycled around by Lucy

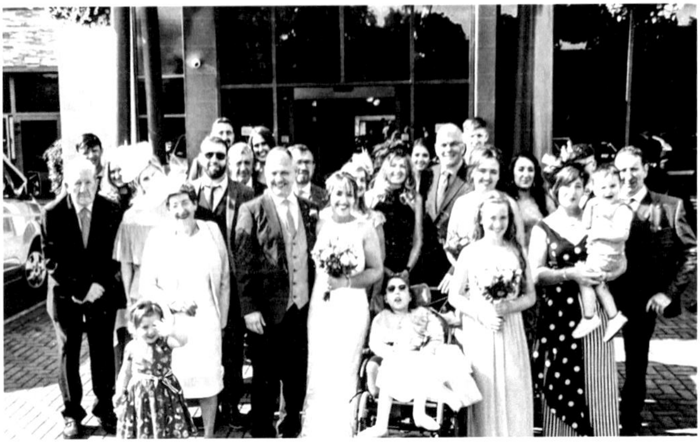

Photo 8 - Celebrating our wedding 26th July 2019

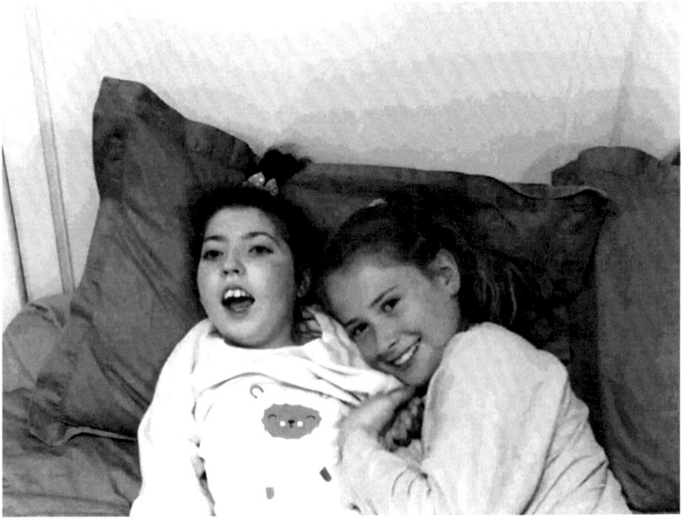

Photo 9 - Lucy and Keri relaxing before bedtime

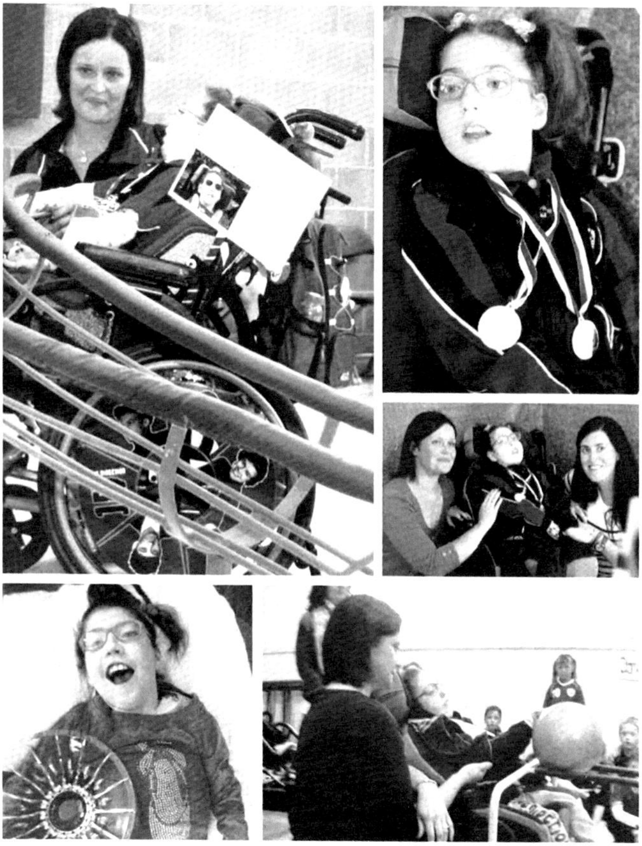

Photo 10 - National Games 2014 - University of Limerick

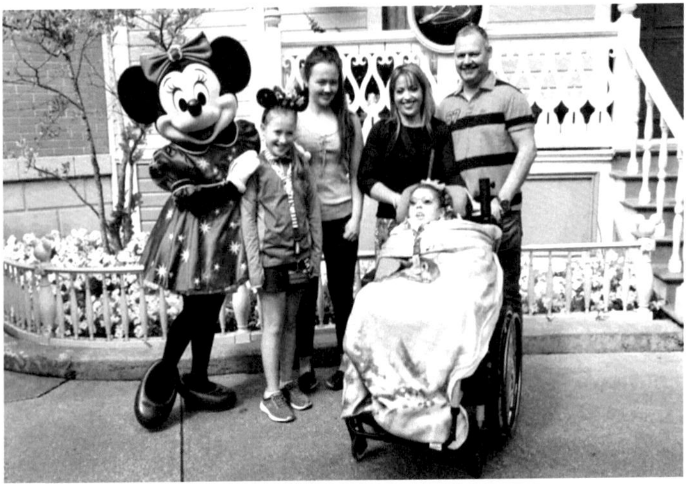

Photo 11 - Enjoying Disneyland Paris

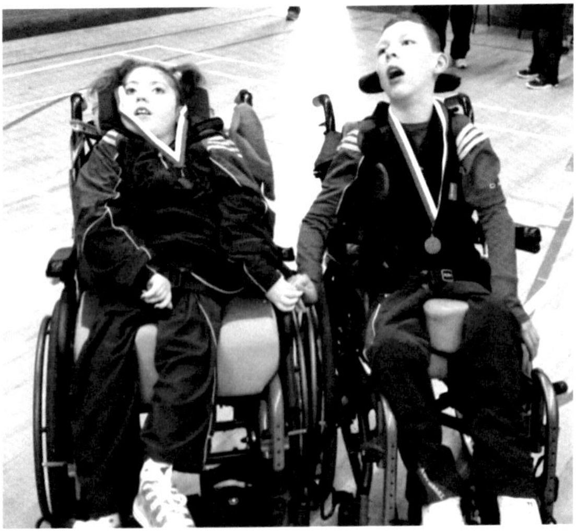

Photo 12 - Keri and her friend James enjoying time together

Keri My Inspiration

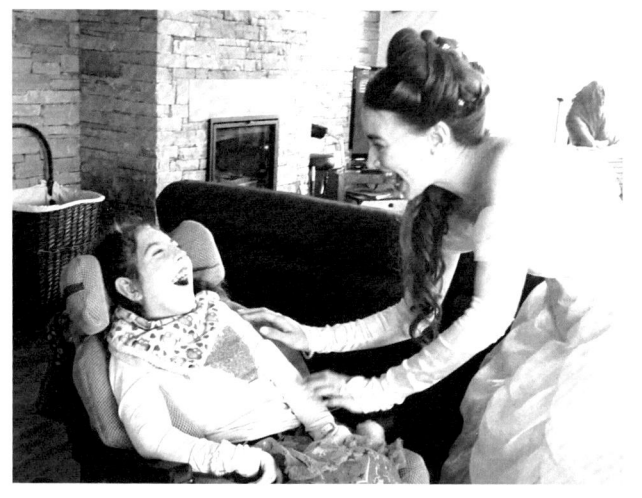

Photo 13 - Keri meet her idol Belle

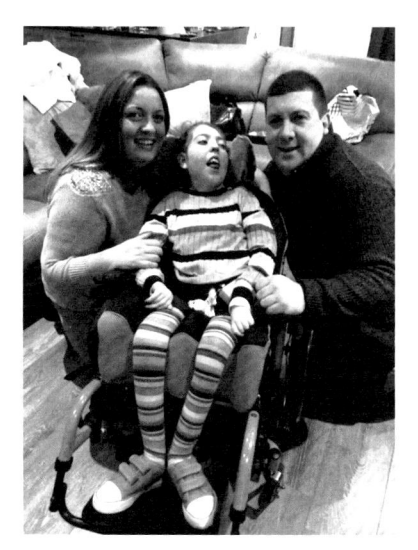

Photo 14 - Uncle Cathal and Amanda with Keri

20

The Dance

The PEG made a massive difference to Keri. She no longer had to expend all her energy just to eat and drink, nor was she at risk of aspiration. Feeding no longer upset her. During the period of adjustment, Keri benefited hugely from alternative therapies of Kinesiology, faith healing and Osteopathy, together with assistance from the seating clinic, physio and dieticians at the CRC and locally. She began to gain weight and regain some quality of life. She could even return to school part-time. By this stage, she had been out of school for five months. The school were absolutely delighted to have Keri back, as was she, back with her friends and her style-icon, Siobhan. The National Games were coming up, and to our enormous delight, Keri was offered a place. It was the opportunity of a lifetime.

Easter was always a time of great excitement in our house. On Easter morning, I always put a trail of mini eggs throughout the hall and two little buckets at the end of the girls' beds. Lucy would put one of the little buckets on Keri's lap, and off they would go together collecting eggs, arriving at the end of the trail to their favourite Easter egg. Lucy would never leave the room without Keri on all these special occasions. On Easter Sunday, she would still get a little half chocolate button or two on her tongue to enjoy. She sadly wasn't allowed any more than this due to her aspiration risk, but she enjoyed the taste, and we all really celebrated that with her.

Shortly after Keri came home from the hospital, Ruth announced that she was leaving us due to personal reasons. While we totally understood her position, we were so sorry to see her go. She had been an incredible support and friend to us at a really difficult time. Happily, she still visits us from time to time and always takes such an interest in Keri.

A very happy family day came upon us in May 2014 for Lucy's First Holy Communion. It was fantastic to have a focus on our wonderful Lucy and to celebrate her milestone, especially after such a difficult six months where so much of the focus had been on Keri. Lucy insisted on wearing Keri's communion dress, a special dress as it was her big sister's. Lucy always looked up to Keri so much, just like every little sister. She had Keri on a pedestal, even though Lucy was, by now, physically bigger than her. We had a splendid day, the weather was gorgeous, and it was all about Lucy.

After the ceremony at our local parish church, sixty or so family and friends dined in Lucy's venue of choice,

Kilcoran Lodge. Keri was as good as gold and really enjoyed seeing her sister bask in glory, love, and attention.

Later that month, we had another big day out. I had surprised the girls the previous Christmas 2013 with four tickets to the One Direction Concert at Croke Park in Dublin. The girls loved that band. Every time a One Direction song was played on the radio, Keri's eyes would light up; her reaction to their music was priceless. I had also managed to get the girls' little bomber jackets emblazoned with 'One Direction' and the names of each of their favourite singers printed on the sleeves. Unfortunately, during this time, Keri's spine was causing her enormous discomfort, so her pain medication was again increased, making her quite drowsy. So it was decided that Cora was to be our fourth party member, and we were just thrilled she could join us. I carefully planned the day and night to ensure Keri had all the necessary comforts.

I checked us into a fabulous wheelchair accessible room at the Citywest Hotel and arranged for room service so we could eat while Keri laid out to rest before the concert. We took a wheelchair accessible taxi to and from the concert, and we were blessed with a fabulous driver who made Keri his priority, making sure we were delivered and later collected as close to the venue as possible. Lucy was so excited, hand in hand with Cora, as I wheeled Keri in, both girls dazzling the staff in their stylish bomber jackets. The wheelchair area was just perfect; it was safe, spacious and comfortable for all concerned. Keri was asleep in her chair, but that was OK. I knew she would wake up for a part of the show and that she would enjoy it, which was all that mattered to me.

Looking at our situation objectively, one would think we should never have attended this concert at this time. Keri was, in truth, very unwell. She was heavily medicated to manage her unbearable pain and was in the early stages of adjusting to her PEG. However, I felt that life had to be lived and that each smile we got from her was a treasure that should be captured and celebrated. Planning and executing the logistics took some organisation, but boy, it was worth it! Once the concert started, Keri slowly opened her eyes. It took her a little time to come around, but when she did, she was transported. Once fully awake and off her PEG feed line, I danced with her in my arms for the entirety of the concert so she could experience every possible smidgen of the joy of it. Lucy and Cora danced too, the four of us together, singing, smiling, beaming. In those precious moments, with Lucy beside us, Keri in my arms, all swinging to the music, we were bedazzled in a flash of freedom. The pain, heartache, frustration and worry of the previous six months swayed away from us with the music. With my limbs swinging us and Keri's unquestionable magic sparkling through her eyes, we were dancing as one, the essencc of strength, freedom, and joy. The fire beneath my feet, as the lyrics go, was burning bright. My girls and I had together discovered our very own heaven on earth.

21

Santa

It will probably come as no surprise that Christmas has always been a mega event in our family. Keri and Lucy absolutely loved it. We went all out on the decorating, inside and out, with a massive tree bedecked with various treasure troves of mementoes made, bought and gifted to us over the years, each and everyone carrying so many special memories. Scoil Aonghusa went all out with the *real Santa,* doing a private session with the children from the rainbow room. He was no fake Santa. It was a magical experience. Santa brought Keri and Lucy many a wonderful gift, but the year Santa brought Keri her bicycle, which I could cycle and Keri could sit up front in her wheelchair all strapped in safely, is one of the best ever. That year, Lucy got her go-cart, which she got years of fun out of. That Christmas morning, I wrapped Keri nice and cosy as I did on the Ice rink, and Lucy wrapped up cosy, too. She jumped in behind Keri, and we cycled up to the ballroom in Fethard, down through the Valley, showing Nanny Mary and Chris and all their neighbours what Keri had got from Santa that we all could enjoy. We headed back up the Valley heading home, stopping cars in their tracks, and we rang the bell on her bicycle, singing Christmas Songs. Now, that was one to remember, one I hold very dear in my heart.

Every year, we went ice skating, and the girls adored it. Luckily, the ice rink in Kilkenny welcomed and facilitated wheelchair users. On our very first visit, to our surprise and delight, the owner generously arranged to have Keri taken out on the ice. I never could have imagined it possible, but once again, Keri's magic opened up new horizons for her and children like her. The ice marshals were great to take her out on the ice, and eventually, I took a chance and brought her out myself. It was utter bliss. Keri's wheelchair was my 'penguin' to keep me upright, and she made me look like I could actually ice-skate! Keri always brought out the best version of me. That good luck quickly changed when I was left to my own devices while Keri was taken away for a fast spin around the rink by a marshal. She loved it! I made it my business to ensure we did as many trips each Christmas to the ice as possible, particularly during quiet spells, to maximise the enjoyment for Keri. I always wrapped Keri up in a really cosy hat, scarf, and mittens and put a hot water bottle under her blanket to keep her warm. I also used a fleece lined, waterproof footmuff for Keri, which I had specially made, a replica of the footmuffs one would use with a baby pram. This footmuff would go up the back of Keri's legs, keeping her contained and warm, with her arms cosily tucked in. This was another thing Lucy and Keri could enjoy together.

I enquired if it would be possible for the pupils of Keri's school to share this joy and have a go, which was confirmed. The school visit then became an annual event, occurring just before the rink would close down each year. Parents, children and staff all came together for a wonderful day out. Incredible smiles, laughs, and cherished memories were in the making each Christmas.

As a family, we loved visiting *Santa* in various venues, travelling far and wide for the experiences. Whether it was Rathwood, Mount Juliet, Kilkenny, Waterford Winter Wonderland or Meadows & Byrne, there you would find a gang of us, Keri's eyes alight in wonder at the lights, the sparkle and the magic of Christmas.

22

Athlete

When she was ten years old, Keri was honoured to be selected to participate in the *Motor Activities-Ramp Bowling & Ball Push* at the National Games in May 2014. I will never forget the morning I was told that Keri had been selected-while I was beaming with pride, but I also felt the tug at my heartstrings as it was announced that Keri would be under a carer with whom she would share a hotel room for the weekend. A couple of weeks later, I was relieved to learn that Keri would be cared for by Imelda Sinclair. Imelda was an extraordinary carer (SNA) who knew Keri very well and was also a carer in her classroom. I was to be an onlooker for the weekend, a crazily proud Mammy on the sidelines. I had to get over myself and my separation anxiety and be OK with that. This was Keri's moment, not mine.

Keri was a busy athlete in the run up to the games. The staff at school put so much work and time into training all of the athletes. The athletes travelled around to various schools in the area, all equipment in tow, to show pupils in the area what they could do and to celebrate their participation. This took a lot of time, effort and planning on the part of the school, but they never complained. All the schools were amazed by what the athletes could do. The support, clapping, goodwill, and hip/hip/hurrays were absolutely mesmerising. I cried so many tears of pride and joy, and I never tired of seeing the performances. It was just wonderful to witness the achievement of every single athlete every single time. So much hard work went into each and every move, and the determination on each athlete's face was both humbling and heart-warming to see. A laugh was had when we realised the national games tracksuit was navy - definitely not in keeping with Keri's preference for pink, purple and sparkle, but we made up for it with hair and footwear accessories to keep her happy!

Keri and James had a really special bond. It was around this time that we decided to take a photograph of them together. We wheeled their chairs side by side and set up for a photograph. While Keri would ordinarily have had her arms pinned in by her side, in this particular moment, both she and James reached out their little hands from their chairs and clasped them. Keri and James were holding hands, with the most enormous beaming smiles on their faces. I cried tears of joy and utter pride. My special little girl had found her prince, and I couldn't have been more approving.

The launch of the National Games took place on Thursday, 22nd of May 2014, at Castletroy Park Hotel in

Limerick. The school had their own launch on the 26th of May, a memorable evening where the athletes performed for their families, proudly showing us all what they could do, followed by a parade outside on the track, where each athlete held or helped to hold the Olympic torch. The icing on the cake came when athlete Terry Ryan lit the Olympic flame at the conclusion of the evening. What an experience for us all!

After much preparation, training and excitement, the National Games event itself took place over three days from Thursday, 12th June to Saturday, 14th June 2014 at the University of Limerick. I was very blessed to be asked to join in with the celebrations and come along to the event for the entire weekend, and I didn't want to miss a minute of it. There was an incredible send-off organised by the school. Not only did the team have a Garda escort, but there was a massive guard of honour formed by the staff and parents from the school building all the way out to the school gate, with cheering, waving and clapping as the team bus departed. Keri and her fellow athletes on board the bus lapped up the stardom while the driver tooted the horn for the crowd. There were shouts out and beaming smiles aplenty from every passenger on board. Cora and I followed the bus right behind. It was an incredible moment, every single second of it so precious. I had never witnessed such excitement, positivity, energy, love, and devotion as I did on that day as we left Scoil Aonghusa with our very special athletes. It was a huge bonus that Cora could join me, as she was such a huge part of both our lives.

When we arrived at the Raddisson Blue Hotel and Spa in Limerick, we checked into our rooms, and I spoke with Imelda about Keri's PEG feeds. As per her new regime, she was to be fed slowly, little and often. I offered to show Imelda how to operate the PEG, and she was very happy to do it, taking to it like a duck to water. She was also very happy to look after Keri's medication, which, when needed, would require to be administered in an instant so as to ensure a spasm didn't get too severe. By now, Keri was going into a headlock with spasms in her neck, which caused her head to become locked to the side, sometimes numerous times a day. She needed to be on top of things to try and prevent this from happening. If we saw it start to happen, we would give her a small dose of Midazolam to break the spasm.

Keri and another athlete, Nicole, shared a room together, which was very special. Imelda shared Keri with me in the evenings at the hotel, allowing her to have her dinner in peace, allowing Keri and I to have our time together and our essential cuddles! Where there is a will, there is a way!

The opening ceremony was truly memorable on Thursday evening, and the athletes were treated like royalty. There was a parade with a marching band into the People's Park in Limerick City, where the music and celebrations continued. The next day, different events were arranged for all participants, including hair braiding, face painting, arts and crafts, spa treatments and a myriad of games. Everyone was catered for. Cora and I enjoyed looking at other events Keri's schoolmates were participating in on Friday. Every minute was fabulous to have Cora's company.

Keri's event took place on the Saturday. Both families arrived-grandparents, aunts, uncles, cousins, friends, Chalkie and Mark were all there to support Keri. I had t-shirts printed for Lucy, her friend Kiera and I with our names inscribed on them. Mine read, 'Keri's mom', which I wore with indescribable pride. Lucy's read 'Keri's sister Lucy'. As the athletes entered the main building, the atmosphere erupted. With music blaring, waving and cheering, every participant got their moment of glory, their families in floods of tears with unbridled pride and joy.

Keri's expression of sheer grit and determination as she did the bowling was a sight to behold. I knew that Keri was in quite a lot of pain that day, as she was still awaiting her spinal surgery, but she was one class act, and people would never have guessed the pain she was in to look at her as she competed. She knew this was her time to shine. She knocked all the pins, which reaped a huge roar from her supporters. The pride on Imelda's face was priceless. It was then time for the push ball, which Keri did brilliantly. One must remember that these tasks are enormous challenges for these athletes. While it may be easy for most, children like Keri find these activities ferociously difficult to complete. We all celebrated with all the other athletes who also took their turn in this event, including her good friends, Joe Kelly, Cameron Meehan and Nicole Hassett.

We all got to join Keri for photographs as she was presented with her medals. There were great celebrations back at the hotel after the event closed with all our young athletes and their families. Having all our close friends and family with us made it even more special. After she returned home, Keri was awarded for her participation in the 'Special Needs Olympics' Fethard Sports Achievement Award for July 2014 hosted by Butlers Sports Bar and also awarded joint winner in January 2015, two more proud memorial occasions with great celebrations. In September, an evening was organised by Scoil Aonghusa to present each athlete with their own personalised photobooks of their participation in the National Games. No two books were the same, and a huge amount of work was put into showcasing the special moments of the games. Keri's book remains proudly on display in our home to this day.

During the same weekend as the National Games, Lucy was performing in her 'On Your Toes' show on Friday and Saturday nights. It was terrible that the events coincided as Lucy's show was also so important to us all, but we managed it well with plenty of teamwork from friends and family. With Chalkie's help, Lucy was able to be there for Keri's competition and get back in time for her own show that evening. I purchased a copy of Lucy's show on DVD so Keri could see it afterwards, and we made our own event of it at home. Lucy knew that her show was every bit as important as Keri's competition. Chalkie and Chalkie's family, along with some of mine, made sure to be there on both nights to support Lucy. My two girls made me the proudest mum in the universe that weekend.

23

Tenacity

Since March 2013, I understood that we had our place in the queue for Keri's spinal surgery and that her time would come around eventually. I never imagined I would have such an unmerciful battle on my hands for the procedure to even take place at all.

As time went on, I continued to enquire about when Keri would be admitted for her spinal surgery. Eventually, we were called for a further meeting with the surgeon in June 2014. We met the same doctor as before. I received a cruel and unexpected blow. He said that Keri's condition was so bad that she had a slim chance of surviving the procedure-about five percent chance. He said that, frankly, with such chances, the HSE wouldn't waste time and costs of the procedure on a child like Keri. He said he personally wasn't against doing the surgery but that the HSE wouldn't sanction such a procedure for a child with so many complications. I was gobsmacked. I thought I had heard it all, but this was a new, all time low blow. I went into survival mode. My inner lioness erupted. I made it perfectly clear that I would not sit back and accept this. I said that nobody knew or understood the strength Keri had and that only God himself could judge her chances of survival. Keri was entitled to her chance, just like any other child.

The doctor said he understood my point of view, but he didn't make the rules. We were sent home. The fire and anger in my belly was scorching. Keri wouldn't have been in this position in the first place if it was not for the HSE's negligence during her birth. Her spinal curvature was a direct result of her brain injury. The HSE had taken responsibility for that initial part, but they were now refusing to look after the dire, painful consequences of it. Further insult heaped upon injury. I was not going to allow my precious little Keri to be flung to the scrap heap like this.

I absolutely knew without doubt that Keri would survive this operation. She was the strongest person I had ever met. I organised another meeting with the surgeon, and this took place in August 2014. For reasons unknown to me, it was arranged for a different part of the hospital. I waited all day, but there was no sign of him. I made it very clear that I was not leaving until I saw him. Eventually, we met. The same grim and unacceptable proclamation was made about Keri's slim chances of survival. I was again told that the HSE would still not sanction the procedure. All the while, Keri was at home so heavily medicated that she was sleeping most of the day. It had come to the stage where no medication could control the pain. Her life was hardly worth living. I sat up tall and looked at him squarely. I told him I had been in contact with the media, via Keri's solicitors, presenting the case to them that there was a little girl in Tipperary who had a brain injury arising from the HSE's admitted negligence who was now being refused treatment for a brutally painful, progressive, life-threatening scoliosis which arose directly from that negligence. Had I been afforded an appropriately qualified Midwife to deliver her on day one, none of this would arise. She would now be a perfectly healthy 11-year-old, living her best life. I explained that the media were ready, willing and able to run with this story as soon as I gave the go ahead. I had nothing to lose in exposing the HSE as the broken, merciless money pit it truly is. As soon as I mentioned the media and my solicitors, the doctor asked the assistant to pass him the diary. I gave him a deadline, after which I was going public. I had no choice now but to play dirty. It was all that would save my baby.

The following week, I got a phone call. Keri would have her scoliosis surgery on the 8th September, and she was to be admitted the day before for the usual pre-operative checks.

Leaving Lucy on the 7th of September 2014, having just settled back to school, was incredibly difficult for us all. I explained to Lucy that Keri and I were going back to the hospital so that the doctor could fix her back and take away her pain. My heart ached once again, leaving behind my beautiful Lucy as we headed for the hospital. However, there was a job to be done, and I had no choice. Mammy travelled with Keri and I, a huge comfort to us. Game face on, coffee in hand, off we went. Mammy stayed at a hotel, and I stayed in the hospital with Keri at all times.

To our great relief, Keri passed all the pre-operative checks and was cleared for surgery the following morning. As we proceeded to the theatre that Monday morning, I felt incredibly positive that the outcome would be good. I knew that my Daddy -Granddad Billy- and all the angels in heaven were by Keri's side. The team allowed me to stay with Keri until she was fully unconscious, which was a huge comfort and blessing. Without me with her in this strange place, Keri would have been terrified. The surgeon met me to reassure me that he would look after her and keep me updated as they progressed, but that it was going to be a long day. I returned to the ward, where Mammy was anxiously waiting for me. I tidied everything away as Keri was to go to intensive care rather than back to the ward after her surgery.

Keri's scoliosis was severe. Her spine had such a twist that it was pushing on her internal organs and compromising her feeding and respiration. The methodology involved with regular scoliosis surgery is to fit a titanium rod or bar to the spine, thereby mechanically straightening it, allowing proper posture, and taking the pressure off the organs. It was to be a massively long and traumatic operation, but there was no other option for Keri.

It was a very long day, and I drank a lot of coffee. Texts and phone calls poured in. So many family, friends and school staff were rooting for Keri, and this meant the world to me. Mammy and I walked the corridors all day, waiting for news. Eventually, a tortuous nine and a half hours later, a nurse met us to say that Keri was thankfully in recovery. Before long, I was allowed access to see her. I didn't know what to expect, but I had been told that she was likely to be intubated for a very long time after surgery and that her recovery period in the hospital would take many weeks. When I saw Keri, my fierce little lion cub was already breathing on her own. Keri surprised them all, already surpassing expectations. Keri was in and out of sleep, as she was very heavily medicated, but she seemed to be doing really well. I was relieved to be allowed to stay with her and so proud when the surgeon visited with a beaming smile to say that Keri was one hell of a fighter. He said he was amazed by Keri. I struggled not to say 'told you so'; I knew it, but I also understood that they had to see it for themselves.

Once Keri was stable and recovering well, she was moved to ICU, a state-of-the-art facility. Mammy was then allowed to see Keri, which was a great comfort to her. She rang all our friends and family to let them know the great news that our little lion cub had fought and won yet another big battle. I rang Lucy myself with the great news. She was so excited that the surgery was over and that Keri was doing well. I stayed with Keri until 11pm that night, after which I stayed in the parent's accommodation attached to the hospital. I hardly slept a wink; it was one of my longest nights. I just wanted to be with Keri.

For the remainder of her stay, that is exactly where I was right by her side. I made it perfectly clear to the nurses that I was there to stay and help. As they were so busy on the ward, I felt it was safer for Keri and easier for the staff to make full use of me to care for Keri. She vomited a lot after the anaesthetic during those first few difficult days. I was shown how to use the suction machine to give her relief, and this was the system we maintained for the remainder of her hospital stay.

Four days after her procedure, the team from the CRC arrived to adjust Keri's chair. The staff at the hospital were amazed that I had organised this, but I saw it as an urgent necessity; she would obviously require a properly fitting seat to use after her massive position-altering procedure. It was one less thing for the team to worry about. The CRC seating team were incredible, as per usual. They knew she had just been through a massive surgery, and they were so caring and gentle with her, ensuring the very best outcome for Keri. We were very blessed to have such a great relationship with the CRC. They always spoke directly to Keri, and she was always acknowledged, which I really appreciated. The Physiotherapy team at the hospital set to work on Keri's post-operative rehabilitation. Things were moving in the right direction. I was beyond relieved.

During our time in the hospital, Mammy regularly updated both families and friends on Keri's progress. As I was caring for Keri myself on the ward, I didn't have time to do this, but I wanted to acknowledge all the love and support which meant so much to us. Lucy was brought up to the hospital at the weekend to see Keri, which was a wonderfully special moment for us all.

Having originally been told by the surgeon that Keri would be at least a week in ICU, followed by a further month on the ward, I couldn't believe my ears when he told me that Keri might be sufficiently fit to go home just one week after her operation. The team were simply amazed by Keri, and they did not see it coming that she would recover so quickly. I was obviously beaming with pride. She bounced back so quickly, which was a testament to how much pain she was in before the procedure, that she felt better just one short week after a nine and a half hour surgery. Keri was again showing the world how amazingly strong and determined she was. My little lion cub had surpassed even the most optimistic of expectations.

The following Monday, seven days after her operation, Keri was reviewed by the surgeon and physiotherapist. She had done so well. I was advised that if I felt confident that I could manage her myself, I could take her home. I couldn't believe my ears. After all the rows about Keri potentially not surviving the operation, that it would be a waste of time and money, here we were going home just one week later! What an incredible girl. Keri's local physiotherapist and the public health nurse were contacted to clarify requirements concerning exercises and wound dressings. Mammy travelled home with us. As I drove home, all I could see in my mind's eye was Lucy's little face. She certainly was not expecting to see us home so soon.

Fionnuala had our house pristinely clean. Coming home was like descending into paradise. Lucy was over the moon to see us; it was an enormous surprise for her. Cora helped out for some extra hours that week. Keri was thrilled to see her again.

Having the support of our families and the local team was absolutely fantastic, and it was great to be home. Dan, the Occupational Therapist, arranged for Keri to have a single bed in the sitting room, giving her the option of lying out during the day as she recovered without the isolation of being in her bedroom away from everyone. Physiotherapist Raj called very regularly to insure Keri's needs were met. Friends and family called to keep us company to take Lucy out and to keep her entertained. Chalkie indulged Lucy in plenty of shopping trips, one of her favourite pastimes! Lucy was spoiled during this time, as she deserved. It took the pressure off me, and it was lovely to see her having time to be a typical child-carefree and having fun. Lucy never complained, she took things in her stride, but I knew she worried about Keri. Everywhere she went, she always made sure to come home with a little bag of chocolate buttons for Keri. Although Keri was now tube-fed, I allowed her part of a little button on her tongue for the pleasure of the chocolate taste. What little lady doesn't like her chocolate?! Lucy loved making sure that Keri had all those little luxuries. She was an incredibly devoted and loving little sister. Keri idolised Lucy-when she would see her coming, her eyes would light up. We would all have been lost without Lucy's huge heart and beaming smile.

Shortly after Keri's scoliosis surgery, I was lucky enough to be connected with my sister's neighbour, Lorraine Doheny. Lorraine had known Keri since she was a baby and happily agreed to come on board with a flexible four hours twice a week. Lorraine was brilliant with Keri. What I loved most was that she treated Keri the same as any other child of her age. She was so funny that Keri would spend her time with her, smiling and shouting at her. I often found myself crying and laughing with her. After a tough few months, it was a tonic to have so much laughter in our lives. Lorraine looked after Keri and Lucy in the run up to Christmas while Mark and I got out to do some Christmas shopping. On that occasion, she brought her own two daughters, Amy and Jenna, with her. Jenna was eleven months younger than Keri, and Amy was a few years older.

They were great with Keri and Lucy. They had great fun together, making gorgeous Christmas tree decorations from flour and water, which they cut, baked in the oven and later painted. To this day, these decorations take pride of place on our tree each year, a treasure of such a happy chapter with Lorraine and her girls in our lives. Lorraine brought her fun to our home for twelve months before she was offered a full time job elsewhere. We were blessed to have had her, and Keri adored her. Laughter really is the very best medicine.

To recap, we had our wonderful Family Doctor, the CRC, our local physio, our occupational therapist, our health nurse, a great team at Clonmel paediatric ward, and the support of some brilliant private Consultants. After the PEG surgery, Keri was referred to Liane Murphy, an HSE nurse for children with life-limiting conditions. While it was heart wrenching to have such a facility visiting us, and we understood perfectly well what it meant in terms of Keri's prognosis, Liane was an exceptional professional who became a huge part of our lives. She was a mine of information and support, and she was always utterly respectful of her patients and their entire families.

Life was easier for Keri after her scoliosis surgery. Her feeding improved. She could now sit without discomfort, and the crying subsided. She managed to get back to school on a part time basis. Most importantly, we could now enjoy family time together. We enjoyed life as much as we could. We took every opportunity to have family days out together. Day to day, Lucy had her happy sister back, and she was able to do things with Keri that she previously couldn't tolerate because of her pain. Lucy would do arts and crafts with Keri, paint her nails, or give her a foot massage, all of which Keri adored. To see the joy on Lucy's face when Keri would shout out at her with that huge, adoring sisterly smile was just the most wonderful sight in the world for me. Mark and I got to have time together, which we had missed out on for so long. This was a good chapter, but cruelly for Keri, it wasn't going to last for long.

24

London

As early as nine months after her scoliosis surgery, Keri started to show signs of discomfort. I contacted the hospital, and a review was arranged for the following week. An X-ray was carried out. The surgeon who had performed Keri's spinal operation reviewed it. He told me that a little wire had come loose but that it should not be causing her discomfort. I wasn't shown the X-ray. We were sent home and told to get back in touch should she deteriorate.

Within a month, we were back in the hospital. Keri was in further distress. The same X-ray was reviewed by a different doctor who was on duty at the time. That doctor showed me the X-ray and said, 'That is no wire. That is the bar', and confirmed that the bar had clearly come away from the top of Keri's spine. He showed me the X-ray, and even my untrained eye could clearly see the bar had separated from the spine. Keri needed urgent corrective surgery. There are no words to describe how devastated I was. Keri had been fobbed off by her surgeon when it was clear as day from the X-ray that she was in massive trouble only nine months after the procedure.

I waited to see the surgeon. I asked him why he lied to me. He shrugged his shoulders and said there was nothing that could be done-that they didn't have the resources. A discussion ensued about waiting lists, and I understood that Keri would be booked for corrective surgery to get her sorted.

Within a few weeks, the bar had physically broken through the skin at the top of Keri's spine. Her back was in an atrocious condition. I telephoned the surgeon to tell him that Keri had a visible hole in her back. His response was that I was to call him when the hole became the size of a fifty pence piece. A fifty pence piece is an old Irish coin, no longer in circulation. It is a large heptagon coin, a whopping 3cm in breath. I replied, exacerbated; 'you can't leave her like this. She is in pain'. He replied, 'Children like Keri don't feel pain like you and me'. I could not believe my ears.

The hole grew bigger. Keri's pain went out of all control. I brought her back to the hospital. A discussion ensued about the waiting lists again. I was told the children were going to the UK, but he wouldn't entertain referring Keri to the UK. He said that it wouldn't look good for him to send her to the UK, as he did the initial operation. I looked at him squarely and asked, 'Are you saying that you are refusing to send my daughter to the UK to have her back re-done because it wouldn't look good for you?' He shrugged his shoulders with a smirk on his face and said, 'Yes, that is exactly what I am telling you'. In the corner of my eye, I could see a mop for the floor. He was so lucky he didn't get a slap of it. I just had to leave the room with my precious Keri at that point. I was close to a breakdown. I felt like I had been kicked in the stomach like never before. I wondered what else could happen, my poor little darling. By now, it was injury upon insult upon insult upon injury. I had lost track of insults and injuries. I was being ground down to almost dust. I knew that day that Keri and I were on our own now as we left that hospital. She was not treated for her pain. I got no advice as to how to handle her without hurting her. Nobody told me what would happen next. My Keri had been flung on the scrap heap.

The clerical staff of the hospital didn't ring me about this problem until eighteen months later, offering an appointment to attend for corrective surgery, by which time, had we waited, Keri would have been dead and cremated.

I got to work making enquiries as to where we could get help for Keri. I took matters into my own hands. Keri needed help immediately. She was in immense pain. Mark and I dressed her wound each day. As the hole grew, so did her distress. My heart was broken for her.

I was shared details of Mr Stewart Tucker, Consultant Orthopaedic Spinal Surgeon in London's Great Ormond Street Children's Hospital. Upon my request, Dr Condon GP, very kindly referred Keri without hesitation. She personally spoke with Mr Tucker and emailed over Keri's files. I arranged for updated X-rays to be taken with a local private healthcare centre. Within a week, we had landed in London and were attending our initial consultation. Mr Tucker was exemplary. He knew all about Keri's predicament before he met us, having carefully read her file. He examined Keri, who was meticulously well behaved during the meeting. I was sure she knew this was an important man who would do away with her pain! When he saw Keri's back, he seemed to me to appear somewhat shocked. Having examined the X-rays, he confirmed further surgery was required. He indicated that Keri would have to come back to London for further tests prior to undergoing corrective surgery. Had he not been booked for his annual vacation, he said he would have arranged the surgery immediately. However, he promised to prioritise Keri as soon as he returned. We left the clinic feeling relieved and confident that things would improve for Keri before too long. I had walked away from the HSE and gone about formulating my own solution for Keri. She had been through too many lifetimes of suffering in her twelve years.

We headed home. Given the HSE had refused to pay for it, I set to work establishing how to fund this corrective procedure in London. I was close to becoming very angry that Keri was left to cover her own costs for this corrective procedure, but I just had too many other concerns to give it any headspace. This lioness-mom had to start picking her battles at this stage, as there were battles at every turn. After a lot of form filling, our health insurance provider agreed to cover a small portion of the costs. I was prepared to pay the balance myself just to see Keri right-nothing else mattered, but luckily, our wonderful case officer in the Wards of Court Office agreed that Keri's fund should cover it. An application was made to the President of the High Court for the release of funds to cover the costs, and I breathed a huge sigh of relief when formal approval came through.

Mark moved in with us just before we went to London for the corrective procedure, primarily to help with Keri, as things were really bad at the time, and I was absolutely exhausted. He helped me run the house when he was on days, and he was a huge source of comfort to have around or come home on those endless nights walking the floors of the house with Keri. Looking back, I don't know how I would have coped without Mark at this time, and I was exhausted, afraid, overwhelmed. Mark kept my feet on the ground so that I could keep the game face on, put one foot before another and keep the show on the road.

Mark brought a new lease of life to my weary body and soul. The feeling of someone physically wanting to be close to me, wanting to be around me, felt so new and so great. With Mark, I knew that I meant something special to him. I couldn't believe, walking down the street, that he would hold my hand, that he would want people to know that we were together. He made me feel he was proud to be with me. I would have butterflies in my tummy at the thought of him coming home from work.

It was a brand new and very different relationship for me. We laughed and joked about stupid things, even on the hardest of days. I could say anything to him. I didn't have to second guess myself. In terms of helping out, Mark would do anything I ask, absolutely anything. He took so much of the weight of life off me as I could share my days and nights with him, and I no longer felt alone. To get a hug if I needed it meant the world to me. I felt safe and content with Mark. He was and still is my lifesaver.

The time came to prepare ourselves for London. We had two visits to Great Ormond Street Hospital. The first was a short few days for Keri's sleep study and pre-operative tests. The second trip was for her corrective surgery, which was scheduled to take place on the 2nd of September, 2015.

In advance of our travel, I sent over Keri's nappies, syringes, medications, PEG feed pouches, PEG feed kits, water and antiseptics by courier to London, an outstanding serivvce provided by the HSE. I purchased fleece nightdresses for Keri and organised for our local seamstress, Anna O'Regan, to amend them with an opening all the way down the back, allowing me to slip them onto Keri's arms after the procedure so she was always nice and cosy. Anna always prioritised Keri, and she had stolen Anna's heart, too. Mark wanted to be there for Keri's operation, so he took time off work to join us, as did Mammy.

It was then time to say our goodbyes once again to Lucy. Making sure she was as happy as possible was a priority for me. A team of friends and family were called upon, once again, to look after and entertain Lucy for the duration of this trip. Cathal and Amanda were delighted to have Lucy stay with them when Mark was working nights. Everyone helped without hesitation. The separation on the 31st of August was just unbearable-Lucy was inconsolable as we departed home for London and had to be peeled off me at the doorway. Chalkie promised to fly her to London to see us for a weekend after Keri's procedure.

Keri was admitted to Great Ormond Street Hospital, and a close eye was kept on her. The team were quite concerned about the extent of her eye flickering, so an emergency EEG was carried out. Unfortunately, feedback on the results could not be arranged in time for the surgery to go ahead, without which it was deemed too dangerous to proceed. Keri's operation was cancelled until the following week. We flew home on Friday, the 4th of September, to be re-admitted to London the following Tuesday, the 8th of September. This was an extremely stressful time, as Keri badly needed her back sorted out, but her safety was the main priority, so I did understand. The bright side was that we got back to Lucy for a few days. Unfortunately, Mark could not get any more time off work, so the following week, Keri, Mammy and I travelled alone. Mark was so upset that he could not be there; he had fallen madly in love with Keri by this stage and felt so far away from her at this critical time. He was devastated beyond words, sending us off to London from Cork airport. He couldn't even come into the terminal as he had to be back to work at 7am. It was an extremely emotional goodbye for us all. By now, there was no doubt, but that Mark loved Keri and Lucy as his own.

Having had a successful flight to London, Keri was re-admitted to Great Ormond Street Hospital later that day. She was due to undergo her surgery the following morning, on the 9th of September. I had told the anaesthetist that Keri's veins were very poor and tended to collapse, but he indicated that he had never failed to get a vein and very gently assured me that all would be well. Unfortunately, Keri was his first. He was shocked at the condition of her veins, and to his complete dismay, he simply could not get a line in. Keri needed a Hickman line inserted (a soft, small, long, hollow tube that is placed into a vein in the chest and ends in a larger vein just above the heart). I was advised that a separate operation must be carried out to insert it, and it could not be done on that particular day. Keri's corrective spinal procedure was again being deferred. My heart sank to my toes. The line insertion procedure was scheduled for the following Friday, immediately followed by the spinal operation all going well. Mammy and I kept praying this would all work out. The staff at the hospital were incredible and couldn't do enough for us. We waited, hoped and prayed.

I spoke with Lucy each day, both before and after school. She was being so brave and so good, only eight years old and a real Mammy's girl, with her Mammy so far away. It was difficult for us both to be separated. I missed her so much. The rescheduled procedures only prolonged this agony for us all.

A complete review of Keri's medication regime was carried out during the course of this period in London. It was decided that Keri would come off *Midazolam*, a drug she had depended on for so long because it was felt that it was drowning out the true nature of her epilepsy. Weaning from *Midazolam* was very difficult for Keri, but as always, she battled through. The medication review was a really worthwhile exercise-fresh sets of eyes made a remarkable difference. Keri was commenced on a new seizure medication. Given Keri's sensitivity, the re-balancing took a lot of time and effort; the team really had to work hard to get it right, but that is what they did with professionalism and exquisite teamwork. Keri was off the *Midazolam* by the time the surgery took place.

Eventually, Friday came around. The Hickman line insertion procedure took place after lunch, with a plan, if all went well, to proceed immediately with the spinal procedure. A beautiful staff member spoke with me at the theatre and went through all the details. He remarked as to how together I was, indicating that most parents do get upset at this point. I replied that I had no tears left to cry. As far as I was concerned, today was the start of another journey, and this operation would give Keri as good and pain-free a life as possible. The anaesthetist ever so gently told Keri she was going for a little nap and that her mum would be there when she woke up. When Keri was asleep, I kissed her perfect little face goodbye and left the room, thanking all the incredible staff for all they do.

After a long and anxious wait, it was confirmed to us that the Hickman line was in, and the spinal operation was underway. I was so relieved; it had been a tough journey to get to this point. Later that evening, confirmation came through that Keri's operation had gone to plan and was successfully completed. We were later allowed to see her in the ICU. To see her intubated was horrific. Tears rolled down her terrified little face. I held her hand and tried to comfort her as best I could. I wasn't allowed to hold her after such an enormous operation, which I absolutely understood. Mammy was so upset to see Keri in such a helpless condition. I held myself together as I knew if I got upset, Keri would become even more distressed. I just wanted that tube out of her throat.

Later that night, the surgeon called to check on Keri and to speak with me. I was so delighted to see him and grateful that he made time for us after such a long day in the theatre. He explained in great detail that the surgery had been a success and that he was delighted with Keri. He said he didn't know, until he opened her up, what was awaiting him as to what sort of hardware had been used and why it had not stayed in place. However, after the procedure, he explained that Keri needed a brand new bar. This was fitted with approximately eight nuts and bolts on each side, all the way down her spine.

I was so relieved that Keri's back was now sorted. My focus was on that dreaded intubation tube. I asked if the tube, which was upsetting Keri, could be removed. He said if her vital signs were stable in a half hour, this could be done. Exactly thirty minutes later, I asked if the tube could be removed. Keri's vital signs were checked, and it was confirmed that extubation was in order. It was suggested I leave for the extubation as it can be quite distressing. I clarified that I wished to stay and hold Keri's hand during the extubation, that it wasn't about me, it was about Keri and that she would be comforted to have her mum with her. The nurse agreed, subject to me confirming I would not interfere with the procedure. Distressing it indeed was. Poor little Keri roared her little heart out as the tube was pulled from her throat, but she did settle soon afterwards. I stayed with Keri until 1am, but I wasn't allowed to stay overnight with her. I felt like my heart was being ripped from my chest to leave her again. I didn't sleep a wink that night, and I just longed for the night to pass so we could be together again.

The following morning, I was back in the ICU by 9am with the support of Mammy. Keri did not have a good night. She had been very distressed, but I felt she was over the worst of it by the time we arrived. I was so glad to be with her, and I could see she took comfort from us being together again, too. Throughout the day, she perked up substantially. Our little fighter was once again beating the odds. That afternoon, her surgeon visited her and confirmed that if she continued to progress, she would be ready to be transferred to the 'skyward' later in the evening. Improve she did, my best girl, so off she went to the ward where a stunningly large, comfortable, state of the art ensuite room awaited us. The set up was outstanding. Each day, a nurse and carer were assigned to Keri, and each one was as professional and lovely as the next. There were a lot of Irish nurses, predominantly male, in the mix, which was fantastic to see. It was patently clear they adored their work, and it shone through to us all.

Each day brought its challenges to Keri's recovery. Her stomach was very upset after the huge surgery, and there was a lot of vomiting. I stayed right with her at all times to keep her safe; I was terrified she would choke on her vomit, so I made sure I was onto her every time she was sick. She continued to show a lot of seizure activity. A consultant paediatric neurologist had been brought in to oversee Keri during her surgery. She continued to monitor her during her recovery period. I will always remember getting to hold Keri for the very first time after her operation. I was almost weepy at the thought of having her in my arms once again. I got a pillow ready in the bedside chair so I could secure my arm at the correct angle. I very carefully lifted Keri out of the bed, tucking her nighty around her to keep out any cold, making sure not to hurt her. Once we sat in the chair together, Keri nestled into my chest as she always did, and we were one together again. She even managed a little smile for me. It was magical, and I felt like we were the only two people in the ward at that very moment. I could not help but well up (these were happy tears of complete and utter joy). I was so overwhelmed, and I honestly cannot put into words how grateful I was to Mr. Tucker and his term and all the angels behind him doing such amazing work known as the 'nurses and carers'.

Mammy sat with us each day, keeping our spirits up and regularly refuelling me with caffeine. That weekend, Chalkie flew Lucy over to see Keri and I. It was incredible to see Lucy, to hold her in my arms and to be with my two girls again, and I had missed her so much. I will never forget the look on her face as she excitedly ran into my arms and the relieved expression to see Keri for herself, that she was OK and had survived the surgery. Lucy kept hugging Keri, and she was just so happy to be with her. Keri had been suffering so much that she had not smiled all week apart from a very small one when I held her for the first time after her operation, but she did smile when she saw her little sister!

I brought Lucy down to the hospital shop, where she picked out a teddy rocking horse for herself and her big sister Keri. It was an incredibly special moment and lovely to have some time together, but devastating to have to say goodbye again after the weekend. Lucy was so upset as she departed, but I promised her I would smother her in hugs and kisses when we were home and that this trip was worthwhile as Keri would come home like a new pin. I cried a river after she had left for Ireland with her dad. Mammy was my saving grace that evening, filling me with caffeine once again and a few wise words to keep my spirits up. Keri and I would have been lost without her.

I will never forget my fortieth birthday in London. It was another day in the Skyward, and I was seeing to Keri's needs. The fact that she had made it through that surgery was the best birthday present I could have wished for. However, it was to be a day of many surprises. Mammy arrived at the hospital with a lemon muffin for me as my birthday cake. It was so sweet of her to ensure it was lemon, my favourite flavour. I left Mammy with Keri and walked downstairs to grab a coffee to enjoy with my muffin. When I came back, the nurses and the carers had birthday banners up outside Keri's room. I was so shocked they had done this for me, especially with all they had to do in caring for all our precious children. I was so delighted that I hardly knew what to say. Strangely enough I was lost for words which is unlike me.

Later that evening, Keri suffered a massive and prolonged seizure for forty-five minutes. Within seconds, a team was around her, including the consultant neurologist who had overseen her since admission. While it was an absolute horror show for poor Keri, it allowed us to learn that Keri could only tolerate 1ml of Keppra at a time, as any larger dose was causing a rash, agitation and seizures. The neurologist came up with a different plan for Keri's medication. While we were shaken by her big seizure, we were grateful for what we learned in relation to her medication that evening.

Once Keri was re-settled, an enormous birthday cake, carried into the ward by the nursing staff, was to be my next surprise. All the team sang *Happy Birthday* to me, and I was just completely lost for words again in this ocean of kindness. Mammy was very emotional; it was a huge and very special surprise for her, too.

A couple of days later, my sister Colette and her husband Steve surprise visited us from their home in the Isle of Man with the gift of a stunning pearl bracelet and, for balance, some incredibly disgusting meat pastries they picked up on their travels. Mammy was thrilled to see Colette, as was Keri. Colette was so relieved to see Keri recovering after her surgery. Having Colette by my side was so heart-warming, as our bond is so strong. We often know what the other is thinking. It was a great comfort to know that she did this for us.

Day by day, Keri got a little bit stronger, her stomach began to settle, and the vomiting subsided. The seizures came under control, and the medication balance seemed to be working.

The surgeon was delighted with her progress, such that he felt a discharge around the 21st of September would be a possibility. We booked flights home only to then realise that this would not be possible as Keri had to lie flat after her surgery. With the great help of my sister Carmel, we managed to organise for her transfer home by air ambulance.

Our time in London was coming to an end. I was quite overwhelmed with the enormity of what we had been through. There is no doubt in my mind that if it weren't for Keri's little lion heart, her strength and her good nature, together with the support of Mammy and all our family and friends and plenty of prayers, I couldn't have managed. As we left the hospital, one of Keri's carers told her how much he would miss her smile. As always, Keri left a lasting impression. I could not thank the team enough. In some ways, I felt daunted by the prospect of going home; so much had changed for Keri in terms of her medication and her back, but the surgeon spoke to me in the kindest and most reassuring fashion, indicating that he was always at the other end of the telephone if I needed him. A return visit for a review was scheduled. I felt so grateful to have met this extraordinary team. The Hickman line was removed.

Updates were emailed home to all local professionals and the pharmacy so that everyone was brought up to speed. Keri was then transported by ambulance to the airfield for what transpired to be a perfectly smooth journey home to Waterford, where a further ambulance met us to complete Keri's glorious and long waited arrival home to Fethard. The reception and ambience which greeted us at home was extraordinary. Lucy, Mark, friends and family, a blessing from Fr Breen, the fire lighting, a spotlessly clean house and a delicious home cooked meal were all we could have dreamed of. I felt excited for the future. Keri was going to be OK, so we would all be OK.

25

Balance

Keri's priceless smile, captured by a photograph taken following a superb night's sleep on return from Great Ormond Street, will always be one of my favourites. This was a morning that was etched in my memory forever. The endless smiles from Keri made my heart sing; she was telling me, 'I'm OK now, Mama, and I'm pain free'. I cried so many happy tears that morning. I was so relieved to finally see her home, comfortable and happy.

Keri's brilliant public health nurse called a few days a week to check on her and ensure she had all she required. The CRC seating team reviewed Keri's wheelchair after the surgery to ensure her maximum comfort. A P-pod was ordered for her to lounge in whilst relaxing in our living room rather than simply sitting in her wheelchair at all times. A P-pod was another chair, moulded to her body shape so that she could recline and relax with her head and body still absolutely supported.

From what I have been told, Keri brought something very special to our community in Garrinch; she certainly brought a new energy and excitement to the area and a new appreciation of life for everyone. These people saw first-hand the battles Keri undertook just to survive, and it had an enormous impact on them. Over the following days, neighbours, friends and family descended upon our home with mass cards, get well cards and gifts for Keri. Everyone was so delighted to see her doing so well. Neighbours like Sham, Eileen and Martha were over and back frequently to check on Keri. Sham would pop his head in the door, say a quick hello and off he would trot once again. This was very normal with Sham.

By this stage, Kym had really integrated into our family. She came to stay with us on occasional weekends and always joined in our outings and adventures. My girls adored all their time with Kym.

As each day passed, Keri regained a little more of her strength. Her recovery was enhanced by the alternative therapies in faith healing, osteopathy and kinesiology, allowing her to live the best possible life her little body would allow. Her therapists were amazed by Keri's determination and will to survive continuing to learn from Keri in every session she attended. Keri would not have had the life she did were it not for those incredible healers in her life.

I worked on Keri myself, balancing the energies within her body, which was shown to me by Keri's kinesiologist. This work equipped me with the tools to gain full insight into Keri's experience of her world, her disability, what brought her joy and where she needed help at any particular stage. It was exquisite work and incredibly helpful for Keri, for me and for our ever-strengthening bond.

I kept trying new ways to bring about Keri's best health outcome. I immersed myself in learning as much as I could about Feng Shui in order to bring balance and harmony to Keri's home environment. I engaged with a fabulous practitioner, Dervilla Griffin, who worked with us in this regard. Feng shui, as I was to learn, is a totally different discipline to interior design and about so much more than just furniture placement and colour. Considerations of this wonderful ancient practice, be they vibration, colour, art and placement of objects, can have a huge impact on one's experience in their home. Every object and living thing has a vibration of its own, energetically connected to all else in the field. We entangle into that energy field as we move around and sleep in it, so optimum feng shui allows us to positively influence our environment, our body and our mind.

We found Feng Shui to be hugely beneficial to Keri. Keri slept better, was more at ease within her body, and there were certain areas she loved to sit in at home. In these areas, as the energies were lovely and calming, she would be at her happiest, for example, when we sat to have our cuddle time-a calm and beautiful spot in our sitting room. Every Chinese New Year, we arranged for Dervilla to visit and review our home, a practice we continue to date with great results. I would be instructed as to the changes to be made. These were never enormous or costly changes, but they did work in healing our home, and everyone benefitted from it.

The time came to take on a new carer for Keri. Lorraine had moved on, and as Cora was also caring for her beloved Grandad, Cora was now understandably limited in the hours she could offer due to her other commitments. Luckily, I was connected to Marie Bourke from Killenaule, who fitted in perfectly with us. Marie and Keri bonded immediately, Marie being exceptionally eager to learn everything she needed to know about Keri's needs. She was accommodating and flexible with her hours, generally covering two midweek afternoons and every second Saturday for me. She became a huge part of our extended family and a very special friend to Keri. She always talked to her, and she never stopped, even when having her lunch or her cup of tea. Marie is extremely gifted with arts and crafts, and no matter what special occasion, she would make the most beautiful, meaningful card with Keri to give to that person.

Marie did such beautiful things with Keri, like enjoying a foot spa with her every week without fail, following which her little feet would rest and relax in a heated boot. Marie read gorgeous stories and played beautiful music to Keri. She brought her outside to listen to the birds, listen to the water fountain flowing and read stories in the sunshine. Keri adored her. If Lucy was around, Marie always included her. Marie has a massive heart-she was so compassionate and generous to us all, and nothing was ever a problem.

By now, Lucy had a large network of lovely friends who would oftentimes visit or stay for sleepovers. They all got to know Keri along the way and treated her no differently than any other child. I fondly remember a shopping trip to Cork at one stage, which was followed by a fashion show back at home in Garrinch, with Keri in the middle of it all in her wheelchair. I had purchased her a pair of baby pink Converse trainers, and the girls made a huge fuss of them with Keri. The girls were so warm and inclusive to Keri, which really meant the world to Lucy.

As Keri had recovered so well from the surgery in London, Mark and I began to talk about going on a foreign holiday with herself, Kym and Lucy. We were more than ready to make happy memories again. In the back of our minds, we knew this good spell wouldn't last forever, so we decided to get on with doing some living. Keri returned to school to see Santa in December 2016 and, from then on, on a part time basis, when she was able for it.

It was in 2016 that Keri received her new sparkly wheelchair from Santa, of course in a gentle glitter, pink and purple, with front wheels that lit up as she moved along, custom made for Keri as the time had come to replace her chair. The dazzling sparkles as her wheels moved captured her and her friend's imagination and initiated many a compliment by passersby. Keri was so proud of her chair; it elevated her style to a whole new level.

We booked a week's holiday in Lanzarote for the summer of 2016. I started thinking about the travel logistics and how best to guarantee Keri's comfort during the flight. Keri had a new wheelchair mould (the cushion part of the seat) recently fitted to her chair. I recalled the previous mould was not too dissimilar and queried with Simon in the CRC seating clinic if we could have the old one back to use on the aircraft. Simon, as always, was most obliging. He inserted a light back into the mould, so it would not be too heavy to carry. This strategy could not have worked out better; Keri travelled in complete comfort for the duration of the flight. Thinking outside the box really pays off in circumstances such as ours. By this time, I had over 14 years of special needs experience, so I was programmed to consider all options at every turn. If there were no options, I would invent my own.

We selected a family orientated, completely wheelchair accessible holiday complex. It was so accessible that there was a hoist to allow an elderly or disabled person to use the pool. Unfortunately, Keri couldn't bathe for health reasons, as she would always become unwell from using shared facilities. The staff were faultless and extremely facilitative; it was a safe and secure environment, so we didn't have to worry about Lucy and Kym, who spent so much time in the pool. We always had to pay more for our holidays, but we didn't mind, as we needed to ensure we had the comfort for Keri.

A few days into the holiday, Keri took a very bad turn. We found her struggling to breathe and to swallow her saliva. By now, Keri was fully PEG fed, giving Mark and I a terrible fright. We had not seen this before. Kym took Lucy off for a walk on the seafront so that she was away from this distressing scene. I examined Keri's throat and noticed it was somewhat red. I immediately started her on a dry antibiotic. Many worrisome hours later, Keri started to recover. We were lucky that antibiotics kicked in fast for Keri, and happily, within 24 hours, we had our old, smiling Keri back to good health again.

While we decided to live in the moment and enjoy the remainder of our time in Lanzarote, this episode really did play on my mind. Deep down, I knew this was a sign that things were changing for Keri. I parked it as best I could in the back of my mind until we arrived home.

26

Prognosis

The reality of Keri's deterioration hit us fully when we returned home from Lanzarote. I contacted Liane, recounting Keri's incident when overseas, and she confirmed what, deep down, I knew to be true. Keri's breathing, swallowing and stomach function were now in decline. A first 'end of life' meeting was arranged. My baby was only fourteen years old. My heart was in shreds, but I had to put my game face on, largely to deceive myself at this point, because I couldn't yet allow the grief to come. Keri had to be looked after just perfectly to her very last breath. Her needs were all that mattered. I attended the meeting alone by choice. I asked for the whole picture. I didn't need protecting. I needed to be two steps ahead of whatever was to happen Keri so that she was always comfortable. Keri was the priority, not my feelings.

I was asked if I wished for Keri to be resuscitated if she was to stop breathing or have a cardiac arrest. An in-depth conversation took place. I was told that if I didn't sign the DNR (Do Not Resuscitate) order, by law, Keri would have to be resuscitated. By signing it, I could later change my mind and ask that the DNR be disregarded in an emergency situation, but I knew in Keri's case that I never would. As much as it tortured me, I didn't hesitate to sign the DNR order. Intubation was not an option-I didn't want this for Keri; no good would ever come of it. I remember vividly how upset Keri was in London when intubated in the ICU after her surgery. Keri's little body had fought so many battles through the years. She was tired, and her condition was deteriorating. I knew that the chances of improvement or recovery were slim at best. She deserved as peaceful a departure from this earth as possible. The fourteen years of experience to that point had given me all the education I needed to be true to Keri's best interests and arrive quickly at the signing of that DNR.

After the meeting, Liane very thoughtfully took me for a coffee. This was typical of Liane's way-generous and humane at every turn. I never wanted to live a moment without Keri. The thought of life without her ripped me to pieces. But I couldn't prolong her time by even a moment for my own ends. It was never about me. I was blessed with the support from professionals like Liane, from our carers, family, friends and neighbours. They carried me. They supported me to stay strong for both my girls to keep the game face on.

Conveying the distressing prognosis to Mark, Chalkie, and our families was really difficult, but I knew that everyone needed to process the reality of things and prepare themselves for what was to come. Needless to say, I didn't tell Lucy. She didn't need to hear it at that point. I knew that time would come, but we weren't there yet. She had her childhood to enjoy as much as possible.

As Keri was now suffering more frequent infections, I brought her to see a respiratory consultant in Cork. Oxygen was provided to administer to Keri at home. I was familiar with its use from our various hospital visits, so this was not a problem for me. She started on a continuous antibiotic, whereby she would take an antibiotic three days a week for the rest of her life. This worked well for Keri, staving off what would have been ever more frequent infections.

I set about putting everything in place for Keri's funeral. Keri wasn't expected to survive much longer, so it was recommended to me that I make arrangements, if there were any special wishes, to go about making those plans now. I knew our days were numbered, and I wanted those days to be full of smiles, cuddles, togetherness, and memories. I didn't want to be worrying about arranging a funeral, nor did I know how long I could keep the game face on to be able to do it. I selected a beautiful princess coffin, with colours of pinky purple and white with a princess castle on it with gorgeous butterflies in flight cascading so elegantly, which I purchased and stored at the local undertakers. I made decisions around the logistics, the service, the cremation and the colours. Keri's funeral was to be a celebration of her life, of her vivid, resilient, loving little soul. There was to be no dark clothing or sad songs. Keri had survived, time and time again, and that, with all the magic she brought us, was to be honoured.

Once the funeral arrangements were in place, I felt comfort in knowing that the endpoint was looked after. All that remained and mattered now was to fully embrace every precious moment.

We moved into the winter of Keri's years, living day by day with Keri safe and cosy, enveloped in my arms. Close to me, she would stay, with her every need met, until her last breath left her little body, of that I was certain.

27

Togetherness

Bedtime became even more precious. Lucy, Keri and I would go down to Keri's room at approximately 9.30pm. I would get Keri cosily settled into bed at a comfortable angle so she was correctly positioned in her sleep system for breathing and managing her saliva. I would then slowly administer all Keri's medication through what was now replaced from a PEG tube to a Mic-Key button and put the oxygen tubes around her ears with the vents sitting on the entry to her nostrils, allowing her to breathe more easily. Lucy, Keri and I would say our prayers together. I would then suction Keri's saliva to allow her to settle comfortably. She found it harder and harder, as time went on, to manage her swallow. Every night without fail, I would then say, 'I love you from the top of your head to your tiniest tosie wosies and back again. I love you, baby girl', as I did with Lucy and still do. I would then commence playing her 'Sleepy Baby' CD, following which I carried out an energy treatment on her ankles to help ground her for sleep.

Keri My Inspiration

As she slept, I would administer Keri with a further feed through her Mic-Key button at 11pm and medication at 11.30pm and 3am. A new day would commence at 6am with Losec, a medication to line her stomach, followed by a feed at 6.30am, followed by other prescribed medications.

Understandably, Lucy started to ask questions about Keri's health and prognosis. She would ask me if Keri was going to die. She started to have trouble sleeping, now more so than ever. She had a fear of Keri dying, and it caused her huge distress. I sought professional help in handling this as I felt lost at this point. I always believe in being honest with everybody, as the truth will come out in the end anyway. However, when it came to Keri's health, given I myself was so terrified, I wasn't sure exactly how to frame things for Lucy. I was advised to introduce Lucy to a Play Therapist. I sat with Lucy and explained why she needed to see a play therapist, a conversation that broke my heart-how do you tell a little girl that her big sister is going to die? I didn't get into detail with Lucy at this time, aside from explaining that this person would help us understand and deal with what was happening and what lay ahead for us.

This help really stood out to Lucy. She and her play therapist bonded immediately. The therapist offered a home service, which was much easier for me and much more comfortable for Lucy. Even though it was exceptionally difficult for her, Lucy made great progress in processing things. Nuala was so kind in offering this help to Lucy and showing Lucy how to express herself through drawing if she couldn't get the words out. This is an amazing service, one which I was so grateful for to give Lucy the tools she needed for what was to come. My baby had to grow up too fast, but this wasn't something I could protect her from. Potentially shocking realities were coming our way, and I had to make sure Lucy was ready for them. In lots of ways, this helped us concentrate on the moment on the little things and help us enjoy them while we had them.

Mindful of Keri's limited time, my sister Colette travelled home more frequently, which I really appreciated. Lucy was always so excited in the run up to her visits; they were so close, and Lucy would confide in Colette if she had something on her mind. Colette's husband Steve, together with Stephanie and Kyle, visited every summer for a holiday, which brought us all great delight. As Stephanie came of age, she regularly visited herself. The girls were spoiled with affection every time the gang from the Isle of Man came to town.

Eleven year old Lucy knew all the names and uses for Keri's multitude of medications. She knew the dosages and the times for administration. She knew how to make up the various formulas, what tablets were to be crushed, how much water was to be added and how they were to be syringed into Keri's feeding tube. She was fully adept at flushing and clearing her feeding tube, monitoring everything closely to ensure Keri's safety and well-being at all times. Lucy often visited the chemist to order and collect Keri's medication-she loved the responsibility, and I knew she was more than capable. Although I never asked Lucy to organise Keri's medication, if she wished to do it while supervised, I never stopped her. Lucy never made a mistake with it. All the while, she would chat away with Keri, telling her what she was doing, what Keri was going to get and why. As time went on, Lucy wanted to be left to it. She asked me to go away and watch TV or make a coffee. She would then prepare everything and show me the loaded syringes before administration. I knew Keri couldn't be in more capable hands.

Health obstacles did confront us in the months that followed, but the team around us were exemplary in supporting Keri. Liane monitored Keri closely whilst keeping in close contact with her paediatric colleagues. Keri was commenced on Neurontin, which was a huge help in controlling her pain. Things were getting very busy. I didn't want to take on extra care as I wanted to inhale as much of Keri as I possibly could. Our time wasn't going to last long. I was exhausted but would catch up on sleep eventually. In the evening, we did a lot of sitting about and cuddling, which she adored. That was relaxing and restorative for me, too, and I could not have delegated that role to anyone.

All the while, my little rockstar continued to enjoy her music, her style and her pals. We loved seeing Keri's eyes light up when we played *One Direction, High School Musical, Chitty Chitty Bang Bang, Sound of Music or Mary Poppins*. She always beamed at these classics, which we continued to play during this time to distract her and keep her smiling.

My nephew Mark, five months younger than Keri, would frequently visit us to spend time with the girls. He had a great bond with both girls, always looking out for them. He would often get into the hydrotherapy pool with Keri, Lucy and I, playing games together. Other days, he would take Keri out on her bicycle and cycle her around the yard, which she absolutely loved. Mark loved to make memories for the girls. He made a stunning project in relation to Keri's life for his school, which, to date, remains proudly displayed on our wall in the hallway.

Lucy was growing up, but she always found time to play with Keri. She invented games that were appropriate to Keri's mental age, allowing her to win and always making her smile. Lucy would often come home from school and say, 'Mum, you look tired. Have a rest on the couch, and I will mind Keri'. Keri adored having Lucy's full attention, and I got a break at the same time. Some days, they would have a fashion show together, where Lucy would take down some of the clothes from the wardrobe, hold them up to Keri in the chair, and say, 'Keri, you would be so gorgeous in this'. Lucy would sometimes pick out tomorrow's clothes on her own with Keri. As the years went on, as the three of us went shopping, Lucy would take Keri away to browse the clothing and return to me with a mountain of items on Keri's lap! All I could do was laugh, and they made me so proud. Everywhere I looked, I could see people beam in amazement at my girls, wheeling around the shops together as sisters and best friends, doing their thing. This was normal for them; they were each other's world.

The time came for Keri to have her first period. Unfortunately, this brought on horrendous seizure activity. She was put on 'the pill' to try and manage it. The pill did not agree with her; it caused her terrible stomach upset and constipation while her seizures continued. Keri's Pharmacist suggested trying the 'patch', which I discussed with Liane and Dr. Condon, which they agreed was worth giving it a try. This was trial and error to get the correct dosage. We trimmed down the patch until the right hormonal balance was found for Keri. In normal cases, you would not trim this patch, but as we only needed it for hormone balance, it was perfectly fine.

It was suggested at this time that Keri might finish school in order to reduce her exposure to infection. I had no difficulty agreeing to this; Keri was becoming tired, so I knew that this would be an ease for her. For me, the prospect of having Keri at home full time was just heavenly. Keri remained a huge part of the school community, frequently popping in for social visits or welcoming the school to our home for regular visits. Staying home suited Keri at this stage. This downward gear change was sympathetic to this quieter, more peaceful phase of her life. Being at home also gave friends and family more of an opportunity to visit. Keri's nanny Mary and her auntie Christine visited Keri a few times a week, sitting with Keri while I got some lunch or did jobs around the house, giving them time with Keri. Mammy and Carmel called most days on their lunch hour from work. Fionnuala continued to help me out in the house, and with Keri and Liam, Cathal and Amanda popped in and out at their leisure. Our house has always been an open door house. The more, the merrier.

28

Belle

On the 20th of May, 2017, at the age of fourteen, Keri celebrated her confirmation. For Keri, being prone to infection and suffering so much with the cold, sitting in a church for an hour or more was simply not an option. Archbishop Kieran O'Reilly very helpfully confirmed the students of Scoil Aonghusa before the service itself so as to take the pressure off these children and their families. Archbishop O'Reilly was very gentle and comfortable with all our special children, and he waited to take photographs before starting the main service. This was so heartwarming and made a huge difference to us all while we gathered together with friends, family, Godparents and staff of Scoil Aonghusa, taking photos together and making more happy memories. After the service, we enjoyed a lovely afternoon in Kilcoran Lodge with friends and family. Keri took 'Belle' as her confirmation name, a name signifying 'fair, beautiful, lovely one, courageous and strong'-how fitting. Keri herself simply loved the movie *Beauty and the Beast*. She manifested her inner princess that day.

Later that summer, in August 2017, Mark and I took the three girls to Disneyland Paris. We knew time was very precious with Keri, and we wanted to make as many happy memories as possible. This proved to be the holiday of a lifetime. We all enjoyed every minute of it. Keri's health was manageable at the time, which was such a blessing. I knew it was more than likely our last holiday together, so we did all we possibly could to make sure we all enjoyed it. Lucy and Kym had a great time. Keri was a princess through and through; in Disneyland, she fitted in perfectly. Her little eyes beamed up in wonder at *Cinderella* when she met her; she was simply mesmerised. I fell to pieces, crying umpteen tears of joy to see her in such a trance, to see her dream coming true. Mark laughed so much, he had never seen me like that before. The game face and the make up had completely washed away. Even the gentleman taking photographs shed a tear; he had never seen such a reaction from a child and a mother in all his time on the set. I was surprised how much that moment affected me, but I wouldn't change it for the world. It really could not have been any more perfect. Dreams really do come true.

Through the years, family holidays always unquestionably included Keri. It was often suggested to me that I should consider putting Keri into respite care to have a break, but this simply wasn't an option for me. I needed Keri more than she needed me. There would be no family holiday if I didn't have Keri with me. She and Lucy were and are my everything. For Keri's part, I don't know what she would have done if I sent her to respite. She was so spoiled and used to being the boss of the house! While respite services are excellent, entirely appropriate, and necessary in many cases, for us, it would never have worked. It would have caused more anxiety than comfort to Keri, Lucy, Mark and I. I would also like to make the point that I totally understand that sometimes it is easier to put your child into respite as the system makes it so hard for children like Keri with regard to seating on an aircraft. Facilities are not available for kids with such disabilities, hence why we used Keri's moulded seats as a secure way of transport on the aircraft. We would be questioned as to what was the nature of the chair, for example, specifications, but thankfully, it always worked out for us. I would like to urge aircrafts to look into this as facilities as these are so urgently needed. Children like Keri are entitled to go on a family holiday just like any other child without having added pressures, which brings more stress and strain on families, which could be avoided. Our gorgeous children have enough to struggle with besides feeling like an inconvenience to the travel system.

When Keri was having a good health day, and the weather was cooperating, we always took advantage of it and got out of the house. Keri loved going for walks around Clonmel Showgrounds to do some shopping and have a coffee and snuggles in BB's. On other occasions, we would visit Dunnes Stores on Davis Road, where everyone knew Keri and where she could relax.

For Lucy, having a sister like Keri came with its challenges, but she always handled things so well. One particular day, when Lucy was ten years old, we walked and wheeled past a lady in McDonnagh Shopping Centre, Kilkenny, sitting on a bench. The lady twisted herself around with a prolonged horrified stare at Keri. Lucy looked straight at her and said, 'I know. Isn't my sister just absolutely gorgeous? That must be why you keep staring at her!" The woman didn't know where to look. I praised Lucy for handling that incident so beautifully. I hope that lady learned from that incident, the 10-year-old showing far more maturity and respect than she, a grown adult. In general, the people were great. Keri was from a small community where she was very well-known and treasured. She was never hidden away; she was known and loved far and wide. I genuinely felt when we were out and about, for a woman who is 5ft nothing, she made me feel 6 feet tall and always so proud to be her mother.

Children always said the right things. One particular day, a lady came over to us while out shopping and said her two little girls were mesmerised by the flashy wheels on Keri's chair. Lucy beamed with pride, so delighted that these little girls were excited by Keri's style. They thought like Lucy did. Those little moments meant so much to us. On other days, a child might ask why Keri was in a wheelchair. I would simply reply that her legs don't work like the rest of ours, which would be sufficient for them. Nothing more would be said. It would just be children together, children including my Keri. She was, as Mark said on day one, firstly, a child. Adults often forget that, seeing the disability before the child, sticking the child in a 'box'. Children don't have that tainted lens.

We were blessed with an absolutely gorgeous Story Massage lady, a one and a half hour session with Mel each week for Keri, which she absolutely adored, especially as Keri loved touch and feel experiences. Essentially, during the story, Mel would use her hands to trace out the story on Keri's body. For example, if the person in the story was running, Mel would quickly run her hands up and down Keri's legs. Keri would let Mel know she loved it-her eyes would literally dance in her head with happiness, and she would smile broadly and shout out in glee. If Lucy was at home, she was welcome to join in. If ever Mel had extra time, she would generously stay on with Keri, without charge. She did this work for the love of it. She basked in the privilege, as she put it, to work closely with my Keri. Everyone won. Keri and Lucy also benefitted hugely from a weekly music therapy session together.

The girls loved it when I would paint their nails or do a little facial or massage on their hands and feet, which brought us all so much joy in our togetherness. We didn't need a whole lot, just time together, cherishing each other and making each other smile. Lucy and Keri had an incredible bond. There was no greater pleasure in my life than to sit back and watch them interact with each other; it was just breathtaking. Lucy would often take Keri aside, take out her arts/crafts table and make something together. She would paint all over Keri's hands, then press them to a page to imprint Keri's little handprint onto some artwork. Lucy didn't care what she had to do or where she had to be, once her big sister was happy, all was well.

At times, even an unexpected brush, touch or gust of wind could bring on a seizure for Keri; Lucy knew this, so it never took her by surprise. She would always talk Keri through what was happening, step by step, gently and patiently, so Keri knew what to expect. With that approach, Keri rarely suffered a seizure when engaging with Lucy in activities together. Lucy would give Keri a hand and foot massage - in ways it was like looking at a mini version of myself. If Keri was up to it, Lucy would set up her skittles and organise Keri so they could play bowling together. Lucy would always set it up so that Keri would win. When Keri got a delivery of new equipment, Lucy would make an enormous fuss about it to make Keri proud. Every day after school, Lucy would talk through her day with Keri as to what she did, what events took place and what her homework was. Lucy included Keri in everything.

On October 17th 2017, we surprised the girls with a new pup, 'a cockapoo', who we named 'Tootsie'. She was mainly for Lucy, so she had Tootsie to distract her when Keri was unwell, as Lucy worried so much about Keri. Tootsie became a major part of all our lives, especially Lucy's, as Tootsie would sleep on Lucy's bed every night, bringing huge comfort to her, licking the tears off her face anytime she would cry. She has licked a lot of tears since our gorgeous Keri passed away.

During Christmas 2017, Keri's PEG tube became blocked. We brought her to Clonmel Hospital, where they worked for hours to unblock it. While Keri found the whole experience amusing, I didn't see the funny side to it. If this couldn't be unblocked, Keri would go without her water, feed and medication. It was a very serious situation. Luckily, her colorectal surgeon in Cork agreed to see her the following day as an emergency case without hesitation. The PEG tube was removed, and a Mick-Key button was inserted. Whilst the PEG is a long tube, the Mick-Key is a lower profile device fitted flush to the skin. It allowed me to change it myself if ever a blockage would arise.

As Keri's health was quite compromised at this stage, we could not travel for a holiday in 2018. Every opportunity to bring the girls joy and to make memories simply had to be availed of, so that year, we decided instead to throw a 'Princess Party'. Keri loved Belle from *Beauty and the Beast*. Keri's music therapist, Amy, had an actress friend who had recently played the part, so it was arranged that she would visit Keri. Well, if you saw Keri's little face light up when she saw Belle, you would yourself believe that fairy tales really do come true! Lucy had some friends join us, and we arranged a bouncy castle obstacle course, food and drinks for Lucy and her friends. Amy organised a one to one session for Keri to have a sing-song on the guitar with *Belle* on the day. Even though Lucy and her friends, now eleven years old, were beyond the age of enchantment by a princess party, they certainly were intrigued by *Belle* and really enjoyed her visit. It was a wonderful party for both my girls, a day to remember.

Music carried us through so much in our house. We always had music on in the background. Keri's music therapist, Amy, came once a week to have hour long sessions with Keri, where Lucy, Cora and Marie would also take part. It brought Keri and Lucy huge joy. When we moved to Garrinch, Lucy, Keri, and I created a routine of dancing around the house. It was great fun, an everyday practice we called 'dance your worries away' with big smiles all around.

By late 2018, we saw some new changes. Keri was picking up infections very easily and having a lot of difficulty with feeding and breathing. I modified her schedule to feed her little and often, finding that if I increased it even slightly, it was too much for her. Her stomach was so small it would have nowhere to go, only back up and into her lungs, causing her a lot of distress and adversely affecting her breathing. Intervals between feeds, hydration and medication had to be very carefully spaced out. We took a lot of advice from Liane at this time, who remained in close contact. Another 'end of life' meeting took place, where Keri's continued deterioration was discussed. At this point, I felt I had to inform all our families of Keri's deterioration again, which I dreaded, but I thought it only fair, so no one was under any illusions of what was to come and also so Lucy had all the family support she needed from both sides and her dad. Anything that could be done to make Keri more comfortable was discussed and considered. I started using a suction machine to clear Keri's mouth of saliva so she wouldn't have to swallow if it was too much for her. I tried not to allow my mind to go to the endpoint. I knew it was coming, but I wanted to enjoy the now while I still had her.

On Friday, 14th December 2018, Lucy was awarded 'Young Carer of the Year 2018'. Due to the high number of entries, she was jointly awarded it with three other young carers. All immediate families attended Clonmel Town Hall, where the carers were presented with their certificates. We were all so happy for Lucy, she really deserved this so much, and we were so proud of her. Her beaming smile from ear to ear said it all.

That particular Christmas, Colette and Steve came home on Stephen's Day and wrapped themselves around us. I had spoken straight with them about what the reality was. Our time with Keri was now very limited. I wanted us to make the best of our family time together this Christmas, as it was likely to be our last with Keri. We had a wonderful Christmas, everyone inhaling as much as they could of our precious Keri while enjoying Lucy's wonderful company, too. Keri really enjoyed all the attention and beautiful memories that were made for Lucy that particular Christmas, especially arranged by Colette, who always took such extraordinary care of Lucy. We were surrounded by both families throughout this Christmas, everyone wanting to make more memories as much as possible.

After 14 years of exceptional, dedicated service, Cora finished working with us that Christmas. She had been caring for her Grandfather, who now required her full-time support. While I was sad to see her go, I totally understood and supported her decision. I will be forever grateful for the friendship and love she showed to Keri, Lucy and me over those years. She was and is one of life's true treasures.

It was the 22nd of March, 2019. I was sitting on the couch with Keri, enjoying a huggle. My niece Stephanie was staying with us at the time. We were all enjoying the moments, as we knew our time with Keri was getting shorter. Mark was fumbling about, but I wasn't taking any notice. Keri and I were having our huggles, our little bit of bliss. Mark came over and asked me to put Keri in her chair. Stephanie wheeled Keri out to the hallway, with Kym and Lucy following. I didn't take much notice, and I just went along with it. Mark put his hands over my eyes, told me to keep them closed and took me out to the hallway. Before I knew it, I heard Lucy exclaim, 'Oh Jesus, he's going to propose!' I opened my eyes, and there was Mark, down on one knee. The face on Lucy was absolutely priceless. Mark had fairy lights, candles and love heart confetti all over the hall table. It was incredibly special, especially so in the company of Lucy, Keri, Kym and Stephanie. I said yes, one of the best decisions in all my life. I was over the moon, calling and texting all our family and friends. I never really believed that I would find this happiness. Not every man would have committed to our situation, but Mark leapt in, head and heart first.

We all knew Keri's health was deteriorating fast, and it was very plain to see. We had limited time, so we decided to get married as soon as possible. The very next day, Mark telephoned a few hotels, and by early the following week, a date was set for the 26th of July 2019 at the Clonmel Park Hotel. Keri agreed, with her glittering eyes, to be my Maid of Honour, with Kym and Lucy delighted to join her as bridesmaids. Mark organised the entire wedding, but he drew the line at dress shopping! That wasn't going to be a problem for us girls. Following a pre-arranged medical appointment, Keri selected a stunning dusky pink and purple dress with matching ballerina shoes at Monsoon in Mahon Point, with Lucy, Kate, and I. One rainy Saturday, a few weeks later, I took Lucy and Kym to Cork to purchase their dresses. Fionnuala joined us. Marie looked after Keri for the day, as I felt a full day out shopping would exhaust her-she was no longer able to do it. In any event, my Maid of Honour had her dress selected! I let Kym and Lucy pick whatever they were comfortable with. My only request was that they select pink dresses, in line with Keri's choice! And just like that, my ladies were all set.

I did one visit with Mammy and Keri to a bridal shop in Carrick-on-Suir, 'My Dress Bridal Wear', where I purchased the second dress I tried on. It was a dress I felt good in, but Keri's huge smile was all the approval I needed. After a few alterations, my girls and I were good to go. Our next chapter awaited us.

29

VIP

Liane nominated Keri for 'Make a Wish', a Children's Charity which grants the wishes of children with life-threatening medical conditions to give hope, strength, and joy. We were thrilled. A home visit was arranged with Trish from the charity to discuss Keri's likes, dislikes and what we could hope to achieve. I explained that leaving the country was not an option at this point, so having discussed Keri's love of music, it was decided that *Dirty Dancing* at the Bord Gais Energy Theatre in Dublin would be a good fit.

Trish and the team organised everything. I explained the importance of proper positioning for Keri in bed, the importance for her breathing, swallowing and overall well-being and that it was difficult to make Keri comfortable in an ordinary bed. Nothing was a problem; we were allowed to bring Keri's sleep system with us, and a hospital bed was installed in the hotel room for the weekend. Keri's best friend Kate Davey joined Lucy, Keri, Mark, and I for the adventure, Kym unfortunately being unavailable at that time. Lucy was so excited that this was happening for Keri. We packed up the bus and headed for Dublin on Friday, 28th June 2019.

Opening the door to our family room at the wonderful Sandymount Hotel was a moment to treasure, seeing Keri and Lucy erupt with excitement as they saw a room filled with helium balloons, goodie bags and gifts for us all. Lucy claimed the pink Make A Wish t-shirt and wore it with pride. A nail technician was sent to our room to paint Keri's nails, something I had mentioned to Trish that she loved. Keri and the nail technician clicked straight away. She chatted with Keri endlessly throughout the session while Keri beamed up at her, so much so I left them to it for 20 minutes, as I felt I was crowding them out! This was Keri's time, so I gave the technician my number and enjoyed a drink at the bar with Mark and Lucy. I was surprised that I felt comfortable enough to do that with someone we had just met, but her energy was amazing, and she was just a natural with Keri. When I returned, the chats were ongoing, with Keri smiling and shouting with joy. We had a gorgeous evening meal at the hotel. Keri decked out with her beautiful nails.

The following morning, I wrapped a still fast asleep Keri up nice and cosy and wheeled her down for breakfast with Kate, Lucy, Mark and I. We had a lovely time together, chatting and enjoying the buffet while Keri slept. Make a Wish had organised for us to go to 'Brown Sugar' salon to have our hair and make-up done. Keri wasn't up to it health-wise, but Lucy and Kate attended and had a wonderful time. They got to experience immense luxury and enjoy the moment, which I was glad about. This was their special trip, too. Lucy and Kate got to have a fun time together, doing something they had never done before. Once Keri woke, Mark and I got her ready for our magical day out.

Before we left the hotel, Mark surprised me with a beautiful gift from him and the girls: a stunning bracelet. I was totally taken aback. Everyone was getting spoiled! Make a Wish arranged for a wheelchair accessible vehicle to transport us to Milanos for lunch. En-route, we collected Lucy and Kate from Brown Sugar. They looked exquisite! Keri was very impressed. The gorgeous Ailbhe from Make a Wish joined us for lunch, and she handed us our tickets for Dirty Dancing. As it happened, there was an extra ticket, so we managed to convince Ailbhe to join us.

On arrival at Bord Gais Energy Theatre, we were taken to the VIP section, where we were treated like movie stars! Keri was taken from me by a gentleman who wheeled her over to a long table, where a huge fuss was made about Keri and the girls. Whatever drinks we required were brought down to us, together with a huge selection of snacks to nibble on. Cartoon sketches of the girls were done, and we had so many laughs. Once the showtime drew near, we were brought to our own VIP box, with the perfect sight of the stage, elevated and away from the crowd to protect Keri from infection. Make a Wish ensured none of us wanted for a thing. The show was spectacular. At the interval, we were taken back to the VIP room, where we were offered the most wonderful spread of drinks, sweets and popcorn.

After the show, Ailbhe arranged for us to meet the cast. It is always so hard to gauge the reaction of people who meet a child with needs like Keri, but the cast could not have been more lovely. They were excited to meet Keri. They were at ease with her and treated her the same as the rest of us. They spoke directly to Keri, telling her how happy they were that she had wished to see their show and that her wish had come true. They said they were honoured to have her, Lucy and Kate there in the audience. Many photos were taken to add to our memories. Our taxi brought us back to our hotel, having said our goodbyes to Ailbhe. We enjoyed her company and the entire experience so much.

Back at the hotel, we had a stunning evening meal. Keri was exhausted after her big day and slept well that night. The following morning, we enjoyed a lovely breakfast before gathering our belongings to head home to Tipperary. The hotel would not take a penny from us, saying it was their honour to be part of the Make a Wish programme for Keri.

This was the first adventure in Keri's lifetime where I had literally nothing to do with the planning. It was all mapped out and set up for us. I couldn't have asked for a more perfect weekend. Each of us was made feel special, cherished and celebrated. They did not just make Keri's wish came true, and they made all our wishes come true as we experienced the magic of hospitality, generosity, music and dancing, surrounded by wonderful people. It was simply perfect. Make a Wish gave us such precious memories, memories that will be tucked away fondly in my heart forever.

30

Nuptials

July rolled in, and the wedding was upon us before we knew it. Mark's family flew in from Jersey the day before the wedding. Some stayed with us, and others rented a house nearby. It was so lovely to have Mark's mum, sister and family with us, as he is very close to them. To his mum, Mark is the 'Golden Boy', which his family agree with, a running family joke. This was a huge event for everyone. Unfortunately, Mark's daughter Kelly was unable to make our wedding, but she was with us in spirit.

The day before the wedding, Cathal and Mark brought Keri's second hospital bed from our sitting room to the hotel. We had a room there for Keri to ensure she had all she required. This room was very generously provided by the hotel without charge. It was a great reassurance to have that room for Keri, and I knew that she would be looked after so I could relax.

I needed Keri to be OK on the wedding day so that she would enjoy the day and I wouldn't be constantly worrying about her. She had an awful night beforehand, so it didn't seem likely. I spent most of the night up with her. I had her out of bed, dressed and beautified by 8am the following morning; she was only gorgeous; nothing new there. She was also exhausted, so I gave her a little medication in the hope she would sleep for a while, but as the little monkey could sense the excitement, she fought it and stayed awake!

Mark looked after Keri while Lucy, Kym and I got our hair and make-up done. By the time we returned home, Keri had brightened up a bit. My Maid of Honour and two bridesmaids were looking fabulous. Mark and I had bought them each a little piece of jewellery to mark the occasion. The 'fairy godmother' organised by the hotel who decorated our function room came to our home to decorate the back of Keri's wheelchair at no extra charge. It was a really thoughtful gesture and the fairy godmother's idea.

Mark departed to the hotel to get ready with his family and best man, Owen. I eventually went to my room and got into my dress with help from Colette, or else the photographer, I think, would have strung me up. I possibly was a little too laid back. She, Mammy and Keri were the only people who had seen my dress.

I had planned to drive myself to the wedding on Keri's bus with my Maid of Honour and two bridesmaids, but Fionnuala and her son John had different ideas. John insisted on driving me to the hotel while Fionnuala would drive the girls in.

Sham, our next-door neighbour, very happily agreed to walk me up the aisle. I have a lovely bond with Sham, and we have a wonderful friendship. John arrived with the car gleaming, our names on the number plates. We got lots of photographs taken to cherish forever. Sham arrived, all dressed up, looking nervous. I had never seen him nervous like that before.

The time came to head for the hotel. We loaded Keri into her bus. I had a little chat with her after strapping her in. I said that she was my Maid of Honour and I needed her to look after me. She had an important role to play, and that was to be full of smiles.

When we arrived at the hotel, I ran straight over to Keri's bus to unload her. I was a mother first, then bride. As I pulled back the side door to the bus, her face lit up, and a huge smile beamed out at me. It was as if to say, 'I've got this, Mama. I will look after you today.' From that moment until she closed her eyes late that night, Keri never stopped smiling. I may have been the bride, but she was the Belle of the Ball.

This was a relaxed wedding. The second time around, one thinks less about the finer details. The focus is on why you are doing it and who is around you to share the special moment. We made it clear to our celebrant and the hotel that this was not a normal wedding, that it was about all of us as a family, not just Mark and I, and that Keri's comfort and enjoyment were the absolute priority. The hotel and everyone involved could not have done more.

Lucy insisted on pushing Keri up the aisle. While I had offered to do it, her response was, 'No way, Mam, she is my sister, and we're going to do this together'. They wanted to do it together for me. I could not have been prouder. The two mothers looked exquisite; the two fathers were sadly missed. We organised a little table with their pictures and candles lit, so they were part of our day.

To walk up the aisle with Sham, knowing we were surrounded by friends, family, and our beautiful girls, really was a dream come true. Mark's two brothers, Stephen and Robert, stood by him, together with his best man, Owen. Everyone beamed with smiles, looking absolutely fabulous.

I inhaled every moment of that special day. Deep down, I knew Keri's time with us was very limited, and this was a day to make beautiful memories to cherish forever. My cousin's incredible daughter Leah sang throughout our ceremony, and Keri smiled up at me for every moment of it. It was perfect.

We had a super afternoon. Keri beamed for each and every photograph, and our guests had great fun, followed by a lovely meal. Kym and Lucy danced their legs off, and Keri managed to stay going and smiling until 11pm that night when Mark and I put her to bed together. Marie thoughtfully insisted on staying with Keri that night in the hotel so Mark and I could have a night together, which really was one of the most special gifts we were given. I didn't have to worry about Marie looking after Keri.

The following day, we had drinks and nibbles back at our house as an 'afters', but it was an early finish, as Keri was exhausted.

A couple of weeks later, my wonderful Lucy started Secondary School at Patrician Presentation Secondary School Fethard. She began to settle in really well there and made some wonderful new friends.

Although Mark had taken my two girls on as his own some time ago, he had now officially become their proud Stepdad. Kym, Lucy and Keri had officially become sisters. I had to pinch myself to believe I had such blessings.

31

Wings

A few short weeks after the wedding, I noticed further signs of deterioration in Keri. I kept in close contact with Liane. Her feeding was extremely problematic, and she was vomiting a lot. She was on one antibiotic after another. Given the feeding difficulties, she was losing a lot of weight and bed sores started to appear on her back, in addition to one on her bum, which had given her difficulty for five years at that stage. Unfortunately, despite our very best efforts, the skin around that wound broke down again and was unhealable. Our public health nurse called twice weekly to dress the wounds, while Mark and I dressed them in between visits.

Dr Condon GP elected to call to Keri from now on, as the potential infection exposure made it too risky to attend the clinic. The suction machine was a huge help to Keri, as it took the pressure off her having to swallow her saliva. During these few weeks, Keri would take a turn for the better before quickly turning for the worse again. She would go downhill so fast she would become pale, lifeless and struggling to breathe. We would wonder if that was the end. However, as soon as she started antibiotics, bolstered with the support of her nebuliser, she would pick up and regain her strength just as quickly. Every time this would happen, it would be a fright, as there would be a fear we would lose her.

From this time on, Keri was on a downward spiral. She never came back fully, and her recovery on the antibiotics was slower and slower as time went on. She was recovering to a lesser extent than before. She came out of each bad turn worse off than before, which cumulatively signalled that her little body was struggling more and more each time she became unwell. I knew Keri was preparing her purple, pink, sparkly, heavenly wings for flight.

On Saturday, 7th September, Keri took a very bad turn. She was pale, lethargic and struggling to breathe. I rang Fr Breen and asked him to come as soon as possible to bless Keri. Fr Breen had been calling regularly to bless Keri, and he always obliged, no matter what time of day or night I called him. That morning, when Fr Breen came, he got a shock as to Keri's condition. I was convinced this was the end for Keri. I asked Mark to arrange for either Carmel or Fionnuala to be with Mammy so she wouldn't have to be on her own getting such terrible news. Soon after, all three arrived. I rang Chalkie. Lucy was with him, together with my brother Liam, Cathal and Kate Davey, who I knew would wish to be with Keri at this time. Fionnuala, Carmel and Cathal rang everyone else to let them know. Lucy arrived home, as did Kym. My heart broke for Lucy, one can never be prepared for the shocking reality that one's sister is going to die. Keri was so unwell I called Caredoc, and a Doctor arrived and examined Keri. It was confirmed that Keri had silent pneumonia. My heart sank. He started her on a very strong antibiotic, steroids, and new solutions for her nebuliser, one of which was a steroid, to help clear her lungs. He was pretty confident he had caught it on time and that she would pull through.

Meanwhile, Colette arrived home from the Isle of Man, and my niece Caitriona came home from Australia, anxious to see Keri for herself while she still could. Fr Breen called numerous times a day, blessing her on each visit. Between all the medications and blessings, Keri did pull through and improve with each passing day. It was such an emotional and confusing time for Lucy, but Kym and our families were so good to her. Mark managed to switch his working hours to day shifts for the foreseeable future until we knew what was happening with Keri. He felt happier being at home at night, as did I, so we could look after Keri together. Whatever the outcome of this episode, we knew well that Keri's time with us was now very short.

We managed to get Keri back on small feeds and hydrated with Dioralyte. We increased the use of the nebuliser, which gave Keri great comfort, the only downside being that it gave her sore eyes. We quickly reached for the answer, utilizing gel padded swimming goggles while

Keri used the nebuliser, a trick I had previously come up with quiet a long time ago. The goggles worked perfectly, and the eyes settled. Keri had managed to battle through this one.

A further end of life meeting was arranged for the 19th of September, 2019. This was our third such meeting, and while at the last two meetings, we knew Keri's health was deteriorating, by now, she was in a very different place again. While the first two meetings were about putting things in place for Keri's comfort, this meeting was more final. It was a horrible meeting. Reality and finality were here and now. I felt like this was not happening to me, that I was looking in on someone else's life. Again, this was a meeting I attended by myself by choice, so I could take in all the information without having to worry about anyone else. Liane and Dr. Roche were again so kind and professional but filled with empathy.

Having Mark working days was wonderful. Every day, he was at home from 4.30pm. I never felt on my own, and Lucy was so good. She had a huge network of friends and family looking out for her, as did the school staff, whom I made aware of the situation. The house was never short of visitors, popping in to check on us and to wish Keri good health. Keri's incredibly devoted nanny, Mary and her aunty, Chris, often sat with her during the day so as to allow me to refuel myself with food and coffee. Between Fr Breen and Fr Everard, Keri got blessings a few times a week.

By now, Keri had lost a terrible amount of weight. She was now almost sixteen years old and weighed just 17kg or 2 stone 7lbs. She no longer fit comfortably into her wheelchair, so the CRC made enormous efforts to sort out her seating as an emergency case. Marie travelled beside Keri on the journey to Waterford, keeping a close eye on her as she vomited a lot on the journey. With her sores and severe weight loss, Keri's chair had to be gel lined and fitted in around her. I cannot put into words what Simon and Stewart's compassion meant to me that day, as they did a joint clinic, especially for Keri, bearing in mind they traveled from Dublin to Waterford. Stewart had looked after all the amendments to all of Keri's moulds since the first day she got them. They did a super job on her chair. They gel-lined it perfectly, and she sat so securely in it. I think that day, they both knew Keri was very ill, so they went over and above to give Keri the comfort she so deserved, and thanks to them, she got that, which really touched me. Once fitted, we headed home, a horrific journey for Keri; she vomited the entire way back, the movement being just too much for her. I knew from this journey that travelling was now entirely out of the question for Keri.

On Monday, 7th October, Keri took a further bad turn. The pneumonia had returned, this time in both lungs. I knew this was very close to the end, which shattered me. Keri had lost so much weight her feeding was virtually finished. The chances of building her back up were slim to none. Colette and Stephanie returned. Caitriona was now back in Australia, but to return again was not an option. But while with Keri, she inhaled every second she possibly could with her as she knew she more than likely would be saying her final goodbye to Keri when she was leaving. Lucy went to school as normal, there was no point in her sitting around at home-nobody knew what the next day might bring. Liane and the GP were over and back most days to check on Keri. While at Mass one Sunday, a lady by the name of Ann Guiry approached me, introducing herself as a palliative care nurse who would be happy to help if required, which I was delighted to know, a very down to earth lady which I liked. Our Pharmacist, Jimmy O'Sullivan, had connected us, having recently acknowledged I needed a nurse to assist with Keri in the near future because, by law, there were certain medications Keri was going to need that I wasn't allowed to administer as a layperson. Keri managed to battle this double pneumonia, but she struggled so much that she never properly came back to us from this episode. My little princess, with the heart of a lion, wasn't finished with this world just yet, but it was becoming much more of a struggle for her.

32

Flight

Liane organised for me to meet an agency nurse on Tuesday, the 15th of October, 2019. Unfortunately, however, when she arrived with Liane, Keri had taken a bad turn, and we did not think she would make it through the night. It appeared too late to commence working with the agency, so we decided to see how we got on for the rest of that day.

I was given extra pain relief medication to be administered rectally. By this time, Keri's stomach could no longer absorb medication, so suppositories were recommended for her best comfort.

Family and friends popped in and out, Mark took the week off work, and Colette spent her days with us. As that Tuesday went on, Keri deteriorated rapidly. I rang Lucy's school to say that Mark would collect her. We felt it was time for Lucy to be at home now. We called both our families and Chalkie. From this point on, Liam and his wife Pamela took over all catering and fed us for the coming week. Only for them, we would have starved. Fionnuala kept our home spotlessly clean. Everyone got stuck in, helping wherever they could, fending for themselves. My priority was Lucy and Keri. Colette kept a close eye on Lucy. Mammy was lost and heartbroken, as was Chalkie's mother, Mary. Liane headed home that evening, assuring me she would call again in the morning. From here on, Liane and Dr Morrissey called 2-3 times a day. They were an incredible support to us all.

During that day and night, apart from when I had to go to the loo or administer medication, I kept Keri in my arms at all times. Lucy had been lying on the couch and sleeping there, as she didn't want to leave us. Once Colette came home, Lucy went down to her bed, with Colette sleeping with her. Mammy also stayed the nights with us in the spare bedroom to be close to us. Chakie's family lived close by, so they went home only to sleep.

It was late in the evening. Keri was deteriorating badly. I gave my beautiful little angel permission to go to heaven. She was so desperately sick, and I knew she had no more fight in her little body. I didn't want her to suffer any longer. She needed to know that it was OK to go. I said, 'Keri, mama will be fine now, we will all be fine. I will look after Lucy. Go to Granddad Billy in heaven, he is waiting for you, your time is done, Baby Girl. Go to heaven. I am giving you permission to go, and I will be fine. Mark will mind me'. They were the hardest words I ever spoke, but I had to give her permission to fly.

Our cockapoo dog, Tootsie, was in the hallway, just outside the open sitting room door. Keri's breathing slowed and weakened, so much so that even as I held her in my arms, I could barely hear it. At the same time, Tootsie became very distressed, whimpering repeatedly. Keri's breathing went on for approximately one hour, during which time Tootsie continued to cry, her head on her front paws. All of a sudden, Keri took a big, deep breath and started breathing normally again. As soon as she did, Tootsie stopped crying and came into the sitting room, walking around checking everything. From that moment on, Tootsie remained by Keri's side. I believe animals are very connected to the angels. For me, Tootsie was sensing Keri was struggling to breathe; she was letting Keri know she was there for her, looking out for her. Tootsie certainly was in tune with what was going on.

As the week went on, Keri was intermittently awake but deteriorating. We knew she was slipping, so we organised for family and friends to visit to say their final goodbyes. I asked that people pray for her to go peacefully so that she does not suffer any more. The days of praying for her to get better were behind us. Tootsie stayed around Keri at all times.

Keri was comfortable in my arms, so as long as she had adequate pain relief, there was no more that could be done at that stage for her, only hope and prayer for her.

By this time, I had not been into bed for two weeks, Keri being most comfortable sitting upright in my arms in our cosy spot on the couch. Keri and I watched a lot of episodes of 'Say Yes to the Dress' that week, our guilty pleasure! Lucy joined us, as she wished, for some of these episodes. Having the TV on was a nice distraction from the sadness. I still could not believe Keri was dying. I kept saying to Mark, 'You know, maybe she will surprise us.' Feeding was virtually nothing. I knew what was happening, but I clung to the tiniest piece of hope.

Liane explained that as Keri was dying, her hearing would be very sensitive, as it was the last sense to go. We made every effort to ensure there wasn't too much noise around her, as it would make her irritable. Mark erected signs on entry to the house and in the hallway, calling for quiet. Incredibly, during this week, Tootsie never barked when a visitor came to the house, in spite of that being her usual habit.

On Wednesday night, Mammy had unloaded the dishwasher badly, which gave us a huge laugh. She had put so many knives into the cutlery drawer that she had jammed it up. In the middle of the night, Mark had to use a syringe to stir his tea. The next morning, Cathal and Mark had to take apart the drawers to unjam them. On another one of these sad final days, Fr Breen called round to see Keri. Mammy was with us at the time. As usual, she jumped up and invited Fr Breen to sit down. As she settled back into seating, she realised, too late, that she had placed her backside on the foot piece of the recliner. She sailed straight down to the floor right in front of Fr Breen. No sooner had she landed than he exclaimed, 'Well, I've never had a woman fall for me before Freddie!'. We all laughed so much. At such a sad time, these simple, funny incidents brought a bit of welcome laughter to the house.

Throughout this week, those closest to Keri visited to spend time with her, have a cuddle and say their goodbyes. Everyone was so respectful of Keri's needs as they quietly popped in to say farewell. So many staff visited from Keri's school whom we consider our friends.

Susie, a close friend of Keri's, travelled up from Kinsale, Co Cork and managed to steal some precious time with Keri in her arms. Keri had a way of making everything perfect, and for those moments, Susie sat with Keri in her arms. She recalls sitting with absolute, pure love. She now says this was one of the most extraordinary moments of her entire life to have had the privilege to sit with Keri at this time. I knew it anyhow from her expression; Susie's face always tells it all. Linda, Marie, Cora, Catherine, Noelle and the family stole some quiet time on their own with Keri during this time.

On a Thursday, Keri seemed to perk up, surprising even Liane, who agreed with my suggestion to try her on just a tiny bit of feed to try and perk her up a bit more. We started Keri on 2.5mls of watered down feed, and to our surprise, she managed to keep it down. Although 2.5mls is almost nothing, but it was a lot for Keri at that point. There are 5mls in a teaspoon, which would give an illustration of how little she could take. We proceeded to give her 2.5mls a few times a day. It certainly helped her; there was a point when she sat up straight, looking all around the place as we were chatting to her. None of us could believe our eyes. We were telling Keri how Nanny Freddie jammed up the drawer, so we had to use her syringes as spoons to stir tea, which resulted in a little smile. We genuinely believed Keri might be rallying, but it did not last. She started to vomit again, and we could no longer get any more feed into her.

We were taken by surprise when, on Friday afternoon, Keri's heartbeat started to rise rapidly. It gave us a fright, as we didn't know this could happen. To gather ourselves for quietness and privacy, Mark and I took Keri down to her bedroom. I took Keri's stats, which were not good; her heart rate was high and irregular, and her breathing was very fast. We rang Liane, who was, in fact, almost at our house. When Liane saw Keri, I asked her straight out if this was it. Liane explained, 'It's not looking good. Did you know that when someone is dying, they often experience a good spell just before they die?' This explained what had happened the day prior as Keri had sat up looking around. Right at that point, with her stats like this, Liane confirmed the end was close. My heart broke. Various calls were made to arrange medication, and procedures were carried out, including the insertion of the butterfly into Keri's arm to make her comfortable. A 'medical backpack', about the size of a thick envelope containing the medication for infusion to the butterfly, was attached to her chair so that it was safely out of the way. I was advised to leave Keri sitting upright in her chair, her head supported with her headrest, as she was quite fragile and may feel pain if she were to be moved. Dr Morrissey GP insisted on staying that Friday night, in case Keri ran into any difficulty, simply out of the kindness of her heart. Those close to us, some who had not seen Keri, called that night to say their goodbyes: Noelle, Marita, Jimmy and Fionnuala O'Sullivan, Buda and neighbours. My friend Linda very kindly gave us some cylinders of oxygen as we were running low, but Liane had arranged for Chalkie and Cathal to collect some on Saturday from a medical supplier.

Keri made it through the night, a night we will never forget. The next morning, Dr Morrissey checked Keri over and liaised with Liane over the phone on further treatment. Dr Morrissey then headed home. Dr Condon was on the way from a trip abroad at this stage, and she called to say she was on her way to see Keri.

On a Saturday afternoon, Liane called to update Keri's medication, but at that stage, she herself had to go home to look after her own child. So as to avoid bringing Keri to the hospital at that point, I took Ann Guiry up on her very kind offer of help. She was at the house within 15 minutes of me calling her. Liane and Ann discussed everything medically required to ensure Keri was comfortable, Liane assuring us she was available by telephone at any stage if required.

We were advised to keep Keri in her favourite place, which was in the sitting room. We were to keep the room quiet and keep her on oxygen at all times so that she would not struggle to breathe. Tea, coffee and food that Liam kindly prepared were available in our utility room. Ann Guiry stayed in the hallway, with both immediate families only, throughout the night. Everyone remained in our other living room and hallway, welcome to enter in ones or twos and sit with Keri if and when they were comfortable. Mark and I stayed with Keri full time. I eased off on the coffee so as to minimise toilet trips. I didn't want to be away from Keri for even a moment.

We were now certain Keri was holding on for her 16th birthday. While I didn't want Keri suffering further just to hang on for the calendar, I began to agree that this must be the case. She put up one hell of a fight, and, as it turned out, that was exactly her intention.

During all this time, Lucy was so good even though you could visibly see the heartbreak in her eyes. I honestly have never, in all my life, seen a sisterly bond so strong. Lucy was blessed to be surrounded by so many people who loved her. Cathal and Amanda did all they could to keep Lucy upbeat; they have a great way with her, and she enjoys them so much. Chalkie stayed in the house continuously at this time. It was so hard on everyone, but we all did the best we could do. There was no right and no wrong.

The whole house was in disarray. People came to the door to show support and bring gifts of flowers, balloons, angel gifts and crystals, which I appreciated so much. I didn't meet anyone, as I stayed with Keri continuously. I did not want to miss a second with her, as I knew each second was so precious. I also knew Keri could still hear, so I wanted to keep talking to her so she knew I was close by. When we were together, Keri was not afraid. That was my hope, at least in such circumstances. Fr. Breen called numerous times, checking in on Keri during those days, along with Fr. Everard.

Lucy came in and out of the room to check on Keri, looking at her lovingly and holding her hand. It was clear to me that the poor pet was hoping Keri would wake up again. Lucy had so much love and sadness in her little twelve year old eyes, it tore my heart out. I was so worried about her; I couldn't tell her it would all be OK. All I could do was reassure her that Keri was comfortable and at peace. Lucy was welcome to enter the room, leave the room, and do or be whatever her heart desired during this entire time.

Saturday night fell, and Keri lay peacefully in her chair. I kept a close eye on her stats while Ann saw to all her medication. Ann stayed in the hall with everyone else when not tending to Keri so as to allow Mark, Keri and I our privacy. Knowing she was right there gave me huge reassurance. Only for Ann, Liane, Dr Morrissey, Dr Condon, Dr Roche, Jimmy and Jack O Sullivan, Keri would have had to go to the hospital to manage her pain. Thanks to all these angels on earth, we got to keep Keri at home, in her safe place, with those who love her dearly. Mark and I were so grateful for this time with Keri. In a strange way, it made things easier, especially knowing she was in her happiest place, with us, peaceful and pain-free.

The clock struck midnight. Our little princess had floated into her 16th birthday. She had made it. All the main family-uncles, aunts, grandparents and the girls came into the room briefly. We gently sang Happy Birthday to Keri. She gave out a little grunt-she knew she had made it-that was her acknowledgement. I now firmly believe her motive for holding on to her 16th birthday was to make sure her anniversary wasn't a completely sad occasion but also a celebration of her life.

We opened presents with Keri. This was really hard, but I felt we had to do it, as Keri deserved to receive gifts on her 16th birthday. Even if she wouldn't get to enjoy using them, she would in some way enjoy having received them. Each gift was a further sign of how much we cherished her, so it had to be done. Noelle gifted her a gorgeous Princess Belle dress, which we proudly got framed, and it hangs in our hallway to this day as a statement piece.

Dr Condon arrived after midnight. As Keri had held on so long, there was every chance she would hold on for longer. I was delighted Dr Condon made it to see Keri, as she was a massive part of Keri's life. Dr Condon spoke with Ann and checked Keri over, after which she had a cup of tea with us. We chatted about different things and our happy memories with Keri. After around an hour, Dr

Condon went home, telling us to call her if there was any change.

At 5am, Keri became unsettled, and she started moaning. Mark rang Dr Condon. While Mark was outside, waiting for Dr Condon to arrive at the house, I felt Keri wanted to be in my arms. I sensed her longing for me as I was for her. I didn't hesitate. It was almost time. I put the pack of medication onto my shoulder and carefully lifted Keri into my arms. We were now in our happy place, having our huggles. I knew she didn't want to go to heaven in her wheelchair, she wanted to go in my arms. She had to be moved from her chair to her happiest place on earth to spread those little wings. As soon as we sat together, she did what she always did and nestled into my chest, towards my heart and said, 'Aghhhh'. That was enough for me to know I had done the right thing. At this point, I said, 'Baby girl, you made it to your 16th. I think now is your time to go to Granddad Billy.'

Dr Condon arrived and checked on Keri. She gave her some more medication to make her comfortable. She didn't delay as she knew our time was precious.

By now, we knew the end was close, as Keri's heartbeat was slowing down. Mark sat beside Keri, and I, and we all hugged together. Keri's breathing became quieter and shallower, followed by one loud, deep exhale and then nothing. I turned to Mark, panicking. I couldn't hear her anymore. I took her stats, and I couldn't get a reading. I cried, 'Oh Mark, there's nothing happening.

I can't hear her, and I think she is gone'. I grabbed my phone quickly and rang Dr Condon, panicked to come straight away. I needed her to confirm that this was it. Dr Condon returned and confirmed it. Stupidly, I hoped she was still breathing even though I knew she wasn't. My precious, beautiful, incredible baby girl had peacefully slipped away, she had died. There are no words to describe that moment.

I still re-live these moments as clearly as if they had just happened. I can still feel Keri lying in my arms. I can still smell her. I can still feel Mark's arms wrapped around us both. I can still feel her face on my chest, her gentle ringlet curls brushing off my cheek. I can still hear her last exhale.

Our Keri was now at peace, but our hearts were in pieces.

33

Release

I clung on to my little angel as the family flowed into the sitting room. Grief echoed throughout; everyone was simply devastated. I couldn't let Keri go. I just sat on the couch with her in my arms as if she was asleep. I wished I could simply sit there, holding Keri in my arms forever. Lucy cuddled in beside us, wrapped herself around Keri and cried her little heart out, the love of her life lifeless in my arms, wishing for her to open her eyes.

My stomach lurched at the prospect of moving Keri from our happy place to get organised. I gave us some more time, then eventually took Keri down to her washroom to give her a little wash, as we did every single morning. I did her hair beautifully, the same way she had it on our wedding day. She looked so perfect as if she was sleeping peacefully. I removed her Mic-Key button so her little body could be free of anything medical. I needed a shower, but I couldn't bear to leave Keri on her own. I didn't want anyone touching her, and I didn't want her away from me. It was a feeling I couldn't put into words. If she left me, it was real, and I couldn't go there properly yet. Noelle, with her usual unwavering support since the day Keri was born, sat with Keri in my bedroom as I showered in the en-suite. Noelle sat with Keri and nurtured her, talking to her and minded her as I showered, her heart broken as well. She minded us both, as she always had. I couldn't even close the bathroom door between us. I had to be close to Keri.

Later in the day, Jasper, our funeral director, visited to discuss Keri's funeral while Mark sat on the couch with Keri in his arms. We finalised the RIP.ie notice with Jasper. I asked him to request that all funeral-goers wear bright clothing and that there should be no dark colours, as this was a celebration of Keri's life. As sad as we were to lose Keri, she had passed on her sixteenth birthday for a reason. Balloons were always a big deal in our house, so we ordered colourful birthday balloons for Keri for her send off.

It was our intention to have Keri cremated and to receive her ashes back the same day, if at all possible. Jasper organised to have Keri's wake on Monday, the funeral mass on Tuesday, and the cremation on Wednesday morning so that her ashes would be ready that afternoon. Jasper recommended that, following the funeral mass on Tuesday, we close the house, as it would be our last night with Keri. This was great advice, and we gladly took it to have some more time alone with our little princess.

Mark and I elected to bring Keri for her embalming in Clonmel ourselves. We wanted her to have her final journey in her own bus, so this is exactly what we did, with Keri in her chair. Jasper met us there; he had warned us this would not be an easy process, but we were determined to be with Keri on every leg of her final journey. I lifted Keri out of her chair and walked to the embalming room with her nestled in my arms. I lay her on the embalming table and met the two embalmers, who were incredibly kind to us, gently taking Keri's hair down and returning her clips to me with a gentle smile so that we could put it back up the same way later. Jasper promised he would have Keri home to me as soon as possible. I kissed Keri goodbye, holding my lips on her cheek while holding her other cheek with my hand before Mark gently put his arm around me as we knew we had to leave. It was a quiet journey home to Garrinch. I knew Jasper would take great care of my Keri.

I wanted to dress Keri myself, but Mark and Jasper said they would stay with me in case, at any point, I could not do it. When Keri came home, I lifted her out of her beautiful coffin. I was afraid the embalming process would somehow change her features, but they did the most beautiful job, and our little girl was as perfect as ever. I dressed Keri in her bridesmaid dress and the matching sparkly shoes Lucy had recently purchased her. I put her hair back up once again, just as it was for our wedding day. She looked magnificent; nothing new there. Jasper and Mark helped me lay Keri out in her coffin again, with cosy fleece blankets over and under her. She had always loved to be cosy. I wrapped rosary beads around her little hands, placed her Claddagh ring, a token of my love, on her finger and placed her bedtime teddy bear beside her. Doing this for Keri gave me great comfort. Keri was my little girl. I didn't want anyone else dressing her, as that is what a Mammy does. I was astonished when Amanda pointed out to me that Keri's coffin had sixteen butterflies on it. To my mind, she had it all planned out so perfectly, and the sixteen butterflies represented each one of her glorious years on earth.

When Keri was ready, we rolled her coffin up the hallway, not expecting to see the crowd that was there. I was utterly overwhelmed by all the people, but they were all so kind, so many from her school, along with parents of children in her school. Ian Wright (Osteopath) arrived later that night, which meant so much as he was such a huge part of our lives. Liam and Pamela had brought in food, soft drinks and supplies, as they had been for a week at this stage, keeping us all fed and watered. I was very clear of my wishes that there was to be no alcohol at my child's funeral. The preciousness and sacredness of it were not to be tainted. Alcohol is for enjoyment, not for sadness. Furthermore, it will only make a sad situation worse. Friends, family and neighbours visited. The 'troops' kept the show on the road, organising everything making sure all visitors, family and friends were fed, watered and comfortable. In so doing, we were able to focus on Keri, on our loss, on Lucy and Kym, and on making sure that they were both looked after. Mammy was heartbroken, and it reminded me of when Daddy passed away. Keri's other incredible grandmother, Mary, was also totally devastated. There was such sadness in the house.

Late that night, we put a mattress on the ground. Lucy and I cuddled upon the mattress so we could stay with Keri. For each of these three nights, we had Keri laid out at home, one of my sisters slept with us on the couch in the sitting room each night. We stayed together. It was exactly as Keri would have wanted.

Deep into the night, Mark came into the room to sit with Keri. He decided to take a photograph of the coffin in case I needed to see it again at a later stage in processing these heartbreaking events. Lucy and I were sleeping on the mattress, with Keri laid out in her coffin beside us. The lights were all off, and it was a dark night. Mark set his camera to capture the moment, all lights off, flash off. After he took the photograph, he noticed in the image that there was a beaming light all over Keri, right above her coffin. Mark was awestruck. He took some photographs from different angles, double and triple checking that there was no flash mechanism causing this light to emerge. I later discussed this with Fr Breen and showed the images to both him and Fr Everard. Both confirmed that this was Keri's pure light and love being received by the angels. Keri was continuing to amaze us.

On Monday morning, I took out photographs of Keri and put them all over the house so that when people called, they would see all the various stages of Keri's life. I wanted visitors to see themselves with Keri in as many of the photographs as possible. I wanted everyone to know what an important part they played in Keri's life. People came in their droves to pay their respects.

Mark and Chalkie looked after the girls, including organising their outfits for the funeral. Although Lucy had just started secondary school, staff from her school very kindly called to sympathise and offer help and support for Lucy. I was so grateful for that.

In terms of the prayers and funeral mass preparations, Fr Breen and Fr Everard were on top of everything. Keri's cousins Leah and Richard prepared the music and songs. I knew Keri would love to have Leah singing her out as they had such a close bond together. They did a phenomenal job.

Leaving the house on a Tuesday morning for Keri's funeral mass was utterly heartbreaking. While I knew Keri would be coming back home again, the closure of her coffin lid simply tore my heart out. Keri was now in the dark, and she was terrified of the dark. As the time for her cremation drew closer, it was all becoming more real. While we had Keri in the house, I was comforted by her presence, as I could see and feel her, but the prospect of her no longer being there ripped my stomach to pieces.

The time came to take Keri to the church. Jasper, Mark and Chalkie loaded her coffin into the hearse. We shared Keri's balloons with everybody there and released them to the skies as the hearse began to move. We all walked into Fethard behind her. As the funeral cortege entered the town, I was overwhelmed with emotion to see the hundreds of people who stood out to pay their respects, many of whom I didn't even recognise. The staff of the local shops stood out, while Keri's school held a guard of honour for her. For Lucy, the local GAA and her schoolmates stood for a guard of honour. It was so humbling and very comforting, especially for Lucy, to see so many of her friends stand in solidarity with her.

The church, decked out beautifully in pink and purple flowers, was packed with neighbours, friends and family, a testament to the enormous impact she had on so many whom she touched during her life. Being such a good family friend, Fr Breen led a most wonderful service and tribute to Keri. Both Fr Breen and Fr Everard spoke so well. Towards the end of the ceremony, I spoke about my Keri.

'I would like to welcome each and every one of you here today and thank you for celebrating in style Keri's beautiful life. What can I say about our beautiful Keri, sent from heaven above? She was absolutely amazing. Her strength, determination and will to live was outstanding. She stole the hearts of so many people in her sixteen years of life. She loved being the centre of attention, she loved socialising and shopping-I have to say I taught her and her sister very well on shopping! Her favourite shop was Name It in the Showgrounds. She

loved the style, so I brought her to the Showgrounds Shopping Centre very regularly; she was a right little celebrity down there, and everyone loved her. She had a smile that would light up a room, and if she wanted attention, she got attention, or she shouted louder! She loved ice skating at Christmas, and she was a pro on the ice. We so enjoyed that as a family. We enjoyed many holidays abroad, she loved the sun. Her final holiday was to Disneyland, Paris, which was the holiday of a lifetime for us. We thoroughly enjoyed it.

She qualified for the Special Needs Olympics in 2014; she made us all so proud, and I was so lucky to be invited along to share the experience with all from Scoil Aonghusa. There are honestly no words to explain that experience, that proudness that we all felt as our families attended, and we got to experience it with such amazing people.

She had a stubborn streak, hence why she lived so long. As ill as she was, she stuck it out and made it to her sixteenth birthday. We couldn't be more proud of her.

We have very happy and special memories of our Keri. Her huggles were like no other. When Keri was in my arms, the whole world was a perfect place. Keri loved the bones of her sister Lucy. Lucy would do absolutely anything to make Keri smile. The kindness and love she showed her sister was breathtaking. Keri was lucky enough to gain a stepsister along the way, to whom she dearly loved. Keri was loved dearly by so many people far and wide. She had a way about her that everyone fell in love with her. Meet her once, and you were hypnotised by her. I feel like the luckiest Mammy alive to have been blessed with Keri for sixteen whole years. For someone who is five foot nothing with no heels on, I always felt six foot tall, rolling Keri along. There are no words to express the pride I feel to be able to call myself her Mum. And I will always be your Mum, Keri.

I would like to thank everyone who has been there for us over the last few days, helping out at such a difficult time. It was all hands on deck, and my goodness, I can't begin to thank all the people who have helped. It has meant the world to us.

I would like to especially thank my brother Liam and his wife Pamela, for feeding us over the past week, as we would have starved to death only for you-we would have done! Thank you to all our friends and families for being there and supporting us and for all your kind words in what has been such a difficult week.

I would like to thank Dr Morrissey, Dr Condon, Liane Murphy, Dr Roche, our health Nurses and O'Sullivan's pharmacy for being there, relentlessly, by our sides, making sure Keri had a peaceful departure. Also, I would like to thank all the extended services that helped Keri throughout her lifetime. I would like to thank Scoil Aonghusa for all the happy years Keri spent with you and for letting us be part of your family. You are amazing people.

Thanks to Leah and Richard for the beautiful music here today and for the guard of honour at the entrance.

There is not enough time to thank everyone. If I have left anyone out, I do apologise.

On a final note, I would like to thank Fr Breen and Fr Everard for this beautiful service and for coming to visit numerous times a day over the last week. I have to say a special thanks to Fr Breen. He has been a rock to me since I was a baby., I have known him all my life, and I am very proud to call him my friend. He loved Keri dearly; he has always been there for Keri.

Also, we would like to thank all who have helped at this mass and the beautiful flowers. Fionnuala, thank you for the beautiful flowers today. You did Keri really proud, and to Mandy Quigley, who did Keri's flowers for her coffin.

Keri, our beautiful baby girl, I love you from the top of your head to your tiniest tosie- wosies and back again, and I will still say that to you every night, baby girl. This is not goodbye, it is, see you later. Rest in peace, my beautiful princess'.

After the service ended, we walked back through the town, behind Keri's funeral cortège, to our home, accompanied by Keri's entire school. As we walked along, passing Dooks, I could hear music, *Dancing Queen* by Abba, but I didn't know where it was coming from. All of a sudden, I realised it was coming from the hearse! Jasper had seen the *Mama Mia* CD, which belonged to Keri and elected to blast it out after the funeral at full volume. It was so brilliant, we were delighted, and I was fully sure Keri would have loved that. She most certainly was our little Dancing Queen. Keri loved the movie *Mama Mia*, and this was one of her favourite songs in the world.

When we arrived home, Keri's school friends and staff let off their balloons into the sky to mark Keri's departure to the heavens. People came and went for the remainder of the day, but we had the evening to ourselves with Keri.

The next morning was incredibly difficult, as we all knew it was now so final. Closing the coffin for the last time and leaving the house with Keri for her cremation was truly horrific. Even though Keri would be coming home in ash form, I knew I could never again see or touch her. Mark drove to Cork behind the hearse, but to this day, I don't know how he did it. He was blind with grief. Lucy, Kym and Kate travelled with Mark and I. Close friends and direct family members attended the Island Crematorium in Cork. I made mistakes on this list, with all the flurry of emotions, and I left some people out who should have been there. This was totally unintentional. I was exhausted and overwhelmed with grief. I truly hope they understand.

The scene which awaited us on arrival to the private location of *The Island Crematorium*, the waves bashing at the rocks, signified to me that my Keri was now free. Fr Breen officiated at the cremation service, saying some very comforting prayers for Keri while Leah sang two beautiful songs. It was a perfect, peaceful, fitting send-off for our Keri.

I was glad that we had chosen to cremate Keri. I simply couldn't bear the thought of burying her, especially as she was so afraid of the dark. Further, I knew that if she was buried, I would probably never leave the graveyard, being the type of mother that I am. It was the right decision for us.

After the service, everyone joined us at a nearby restaurant for dinner. While it was good to see everyone, I just longed to be back in the crematorium, to be back close to Keri. I worked as hard as I ever had to keep the game face on. I was afraid to delve into my thoughts, as I knew I would irretrievably break down if I did. I wanted to keep the depths of my grief private; I wanted to make Keri proud, and I didn't want to upset our guests. At the same time, it was lovely to reminisce on our wonderful memories. Eventually, the time came when we could go back to the crematorium to collect Keri's ashes. Lucy, Kym, Kate and I each got a necklace containing some of her ashes. We were given her ashes in a small box, a tiny version of Keri's coffin with butterflies on it. Jasper organised for some of Keri's ashes to be dispersed into a number of different urns to share her ashes with aunts, uncles, parents and grandparents. When we got home later that evening, we asked our families to the house and surprised them with these urns, beautifully presented in a velvet box. They so deserved them, being so close to us all and so good to Keri throughout her life.

Sitting in our usual snuggle spot without Keri in my arms that evening was one of the most painful experiences in my life to date. I was proud of her wonderful send-off, but my heart was ripped out of my chest. I cried and cried until my tears ran dry.

34

Healing

Nothing could have prepared me for the emptiness which enveloped me after the funeral. It was like going off the edge of a cliff. When Keri was alive, particularly in the latter years, there wasn't a moment to spare; there were so many jobs to do: administering medication, oxygen, feeds, suctioning, positioning, physiotherapy, showering, personal hygiene and, of course, the essential huggles. Throughout each night, I suctioned, observed, medicated and changed Keri. She depended on me for everything. My days and nights went from all systems, senses, and services, by day and by night, to nothing. It was suggested at one stage that I commence antidepressant medication, but I couldn't fathom it, having always managed during Keri's life without it. I didn't want to stop or dampen out the pain only to have to deal with it again at a later stage. I kept as busy as I could, and I reached out for reiki and acupuncture for my healing. Alternative therapies have been my support, and this continues to date.

On the 1st of October 2019, I hardly had time to shower and apply the game face. By the 31st of October

2019, my days had become a vacuum. My soul was hollow without Keri. My heart had shattered into a million pieces.

It is often said that the loss of a child is the cruelest blow. I can say first hand that it is truly horrendous, and I cannot imagine anything worse. Keri and I had an indescribable connection. I needed her just as much as she needed me, if not more. She was my world, she and her sister Lucy. Keri was in my head 24/7. I listened out for every breath she took, every facial expression, be it a smile or a grimace, every ounce of body language, all of which would tell me how Keri was doing. There wasn't a breath I took in the sixteen years that wasn't for her and Lucy and because of her and Lucy.

Without her, my reason for being, I was lost. I felt I was in a nightmare and that I would eventually wake up. I often felt I was looking in on myself, as a third party, looking in on someone else's life. In the midst of my anguish and despair, mindless folk remarked, *'Your cross is gone now'*, *'You can have a life now'*. *'Well, are you over your trauma?'*. I was also asked, shortly after Keri's funeral, *'When are you going to go and get a job for yourself?'* Another person equated my loss to that of his old dog, who had died a dozen years prior. I found myself at a loss as to how to respond at times to these heartless and thoughtless remarks, and I was never, ever one to be lost for words. I cannot 'move on' or 'get over' my daughter's death.

There is no getting away from the loss and the grief, there is only figuring out a way of living with it, and finding new coping mechanisms. Hurtful comments like these poured salt into my open wounds.

The most cruel of remarks cast my way must have been those in relation to Keri's house, where we continue to reside. *'Well, she left you a fine house anyway'.* I cannot fathom how anyone could consider this an appropriate thing to say to a grieving mother. What parent would swap their child for a nice house? I would rather live in a derelict caravan with Keri, happy and healthy, running around me, rather than where I now find myself. My response was simply to say that I pity those people's children that their parents can somehow put a value on a child's life.

I have a constant pain in my chest and an ache in my heart, and it never goes away. Nights are so difficult as I struggle to sleep. After sixteen years of monitoring, observing, and seeing Keri all through the night, my body struggles to adjust to this new life without such responsibilities. I dread the evenings, as I know the night-hours, alone with my sadness, await me. As I settle into bed, I pull Keri's vest across my neck for what feels like the closest I can get to a hug with her. I breathe in her scent, deep into my core, where I truly believe a piece of her resides.

When morning eventually comes, my first thought is Keri, and my heart breaks again as I realise she is no longer here. After unsettled nights of tossing and turning, I always start the day exhausted, feeling physically and emotionally beaten up. I think of Lucy and pull myself together, grab a coffee and paint on the game face. When I gave her permission to go to heaven, I promised Keri I would be OK, so I must keep my side of the bargain. After a shower and a few coffees, I am back in my 'sensible' space and I thank God for having Lucy.

I present to the world as a well-dressed, made-up person who appears to have all the ducks in a row. But I am leading a double life with this grief; behind that façade of heeled boots, lipstick, and blusher is a heart completely shattered. It can be the loneliest of places.

Lucy has lost her best friend, her big sister, and her heart is broken into a million pieces that, unfortunately, I cannot fix. Mums are supposed to be able to fix everything, but this is one thing I cannot fix. No one sees to this day how broken Lucy is, and she misses her sister unbearably. She is now an only child, which she hates. Lucy always has a smile for everyone, but there are days she just cannot smile. She is just so sad, and the tears flow relentlessly, and all I can do is hold her and comfort her, but I cannot take her pain away. The loss for Lucy is tremendous. No words can describe it. I am just so grateful she has such amazing friends who are always there for her, and for that, I thank each and every one of you.

Covid was a relief. It couldn't have come at a better time for me. I no longer had to meet people. Although many were and are kindness personified, those who felt entitled to cast their cruel opinions at me were no longer on my path. It allowed me to have time for myself to feel what I would feel. It gave Lucy and I plenty of wanted and needed time together. We did things we could never do before. The world was no longer a race. We sat together, having a drink in the sunshine in our garden, chatting, laughing and crying together. We remembered our happy and sad times with Keri, and we worked through things together. During this time, I got some lovely messages, cards and exchanges, and I spent a lovely time sitting outdoors with neighbours, family, and friends. During a time of such immense global suffering, in my world, it was a time of healing.

As much as I miss Keri and wish I could hold her in my arms again, I could not fathom having her back if she were to be in the pain she endured for a further second. Despite my agonising grief, I feel huge gratitude that Keri is now pain free, dancing in heaven with her sparkly shoes and glittery princess dress. On the bad days, when I break down in my grief, I will always find Tootsie by my side. I really believe that a little bit of Keri stayed with her. She always finds me, cuddles into me and comforts me in the difficult moments, and it almost feels as if it's Keri doing it.

During the summer of 2020, Lucy, Mark and I dedicated a part of our garden in memory of Keri. This was done by a local tradesman, Dermot O'Meara, to absolute perfection. It has a landscaped path leading from the house towards a stunning centrepiece. A four-season tree is planted in its centre, gifted to us by Keri's cousin and friend Leah and her Parents, Declan and Noelle Cullinan and surrounded by beautiful shrubs, flowers and a garden bench to both sides. A *Minnie Mouse* monument sits as the centrepiece, engraved with the words lovingly composed by Lucy; *'One smile can't change the world, but your smile changed ours'*. Over the base, we have a butterfly image engraved with the words, *'Our beautiful Keri who made this world a brighter and a better place'*. We consider this area our happy place. It is where we can take some time out to remember Keri and all our happy, magical memories. A resident fox in our garden visits Keri's garden every night like a vigil. He saunters in, trots over the stones, looks around and turns back on his track to go about his business again. It is almost like he is saluting her as he visits her special and sacred space.

I had a fantastic life when Keri was alive. We lived for each other. I accept that when she passed, it was her time to go. Nobody on earth could have battled as hard as Keri did, there was no more fight left in her. Keri was perfect just as she was, and she was no trouble, hassle or burden to me. She was no 'cross'. She could not have been more perfect, and she was my absolute universe, as is Lucy. I absolutely love talking about Keri, and it gives me huge comfort. I find myself disappointed if she is excluded from a conversation. Keri's sixteen years were hard on us all, but I would not have changed a thing. Even on the toughest of days, I never wavered in my gratitude that Keri had lived. I knew I was so lucky. I lost my first baby, but I didn't lose Keri. For that, I always felt immensely grateful, primarily to her, for never giving up despite all the enormous challenges. Keri and Lucy are my greatest gifts and my very best life achievements.

My very special friendship with Fr Breen and my faith in God gives me great comfort, but I cannot, since Keri died, face going back to mass. It is just too hard. I have attended on a few occasions, but it took all of my power to keep it together, and once back in the car, the tears were uncontrollable. I feel the loss so acutely in our church. I have explained to Fr Breen and Fr Everard where I am coming from, and they understand entirely. Some day, I might be able to go back to mass, but for now, my visits there are in my memories of those happy weekend mass attendances with my girls.

I go forward now with my wonderful Lucy and devoted husband Mark by my side, my heart aching for Keri but with no regrets whatsoever. The Davey girls and Jack are always close by and so good to Lucy. They remain an integral part of our family, my adopted children. My Godchild Kaycie is also like a sister to Lucy, always looking out for her, which brings us great comfort. Lucy's friends visit on a regular basis, which I love as it brings a nice life to the house.

I am now a Reiki master practitioner and already up and running with my new therapy business, 'Reiki by Clodagh', equipped each and every day with the inspiration I draw from Keri's strength, courage and love. My treatments to clients are by us both, and the feedback so far has been amazing. Keri is close to me. She is helping me put one foot in front of the other and enhance my life through Reiki. It brings me so much comfort knowing I am helping so many people through Reiki Healing and I truly connect with people to enhance their lives for the better.

Keri had her departure planned to perfection. She waited to see me happily married to Mark, to see her gorgeous little sister settle into secondary school. She waited until her sixteenth birthday to pass, so her anniversary would always be her heavenly birthday, a time for celebration. She waited until I was holding her to take her last breath, knowing full sure it was the happiest place for us both.

Keri had a horrific entry into the world, but she healed it with her beautiful, tranquil departure. Keri was at peace; her work was done, and she was ready to glide out of that wheelchair to join up with the angels for a dance. Some fine day, when my time here is through, I will enter into that dance. Keri and I will dance again together, just like we did on earth, she in my arms, with her sparkles, her curls, her enchanting eyes, and her intoxicating smile. I will hold her close, inhale her heavenly scent and feel complete once again. Keri was perfect. She was pure love. She was my inspiration. She brought out the very best in me.

My baby girl lived, and boy, how we lived.

The End

Words of Appreciation

Keri's life would have been nothing as comfortable, fulfilling, or joyful were it not for the incredible people we encountered, on a personal and professional level, throughout the years. All three extended families, mine, Chalkie's and Mark's side, were simply exemplary, and I cannot thank them enough. The neighbours in Garrinch cast a cloak of support around us, support that continues to date. My dearest friends Noelle, Sharon, Marita and Riobárd (Buda) have been a support to me ever before Keri was born, since her arrival and indeed ever since. They have always been by my side. The professionals we encountered from every discipline were and are the world's most special people. While parents like me do not get a choice, these people choose to work in this area and do it with open hearts, intelligence, and compassion. Towards the end of her life, were it not for the dedication and hard work of a number of very special people, Keri would not have died at home in the peace and comfort she truly deserved. For this and all the care, love and support Keri received throughout her life, I will be forever comforted and immensely grateful.

A very special thank you to all the following for their kindness, support and devotion to Keri and all our family throughout the years and since Keri passed:

- Medical, support, administration and housekeeping staff of Rocklow Medical Centre, Fethard, Co. Tipperary;
- Medical, support, administration and housekeeping staff of the paediatric ward of South Tipperary General Hospital, Clonmel, Co. Tipperary;
- HSE Public Health Nurses, dentists, therapists, administrative and support staff in Clonmel and Fethard, Co. Tipperary;
- Jimmy and Jack O'Sullivan, Pharmacists, Jimmy's wife, Fionnuala, together with all the staff of O'Sullivan Pharmacy, Fethard, Co. Tipperary;
- Medical, support, administration and housekeeping staff of the private clinic and paediatric ward of Waterford Regional Hospital;
- Medical, support, administration and housekeeping staff of the Central Remedial Clinic (CRC) in Waterford and Clontarf;
- Medical, support, administration and housekeeping staff of the private clinic and paediatric ward of the Bons Secours Hospital, Cork;
- Medical, support, administration and housekeeping staff of the private clinic and paediatric ward of Cork University Hospital;

- Nurse Liane Murphy, HSE Nurse for children with life-limiting conditions; Medical, support, administration and housekeeping staff of the Affidea Clinic, Dean Street, Kilkenny;
- Mr Tucker, Orthopaedic Surgeon and medical, support, administration and housekeeping staff of the private clinic and paediatric ward of Great Ormond Street Hospital, London;
- Medical, support, administration and housekeeping staff of the private clinic and paediatric ward of the Wellington Hospital, London;
- Medical, support, administration and housekeeping staff of the extended hospitals;
- Keri's home carers-Cora Breen, Ruth Higgins, Lorraine Doheny, Marie Bourke;
- Pupils, therapists, teaching and support staff of Lus na Greine;
- Pupils, therapists, teaching and support staff of Scoil Aonghusa;
- Ian Wright, Osteopath, together with his team, in Clonmel;
- Patrick Power, Osteopath, Dungarvan;
- Liam Whelan, Reiki practitioner, Mullinahone, Co. Tipperary;
- Management, Nurses and staff of the Jack & Jill Foundation;
- Nurse Ann Guiry, Fethard Co. Tipperary;

- Solicitors, support staff and experts retained through Cantillons Solicitors Cork; Liam Riedy SC, Oonah McCrann SC and John Lucey SC; John O'Dea (Wards of Court Officer) and all the team at the Office of the Wards of Court, Dublin;
- Tony O'Keeffe, Engineer, Cork;
- Fiana Barry, Occupational Therapist, Cork;
- Mark Collins and Stephen Brennan of CBA Architecture, Cork;
- John Stokes, Auctioneer, Fethard;
- MMD Construction, Cork;
- Conor Fleming Opticians, Clonmel;
- Fr Tom Breen and Fr Liam Everard, Church of the Holy Trinity, Fethard, Co Tipperary;
- Anna O'Regan, Seamstress, Killenaule, Co. Tipperary;
- Dervilla Griffin, Feng Shui therapist, Cork;
- Stephanie Johnson, Hairdresser, Monroe, Co. Tipperary;
- Mel Kelly, Story Massage Therapist, Co. Tipperary;
- Amy Hill, Music Therapist, Co. Tipperary;
- Dermot O'Meara, General Contractor, Fethard, Co Tipperary;
- Make A Wish Foundation;
- Vincent (Jasper) Murphy, Funeral Director, Fethard, Co. Tipperary;

- Management and staff at The Clonmel Park Hotel (Talbot Hotel), Poppyfields, Clonmel;
- Management and staff at the Hotel Minella, Clonmel, Co. Tipperary;
- Everybody who was so supportive of Lucy over the years, including staff and families of the Holy Trinity National School, Fethard and the Patrician Presentation Secondary School, Fethard.
- My dearest Dr. Eddie McGrath, my deepest appreciation for all you did, for my gorgeous Keri and us as a family, always in my heart RIP.

Please Review

Dear reader,

Thank you for taking the time to read this book. I would really appreciate if you could spread the word about it and if you purchased it online, if you would leave a review.

Thank You,

Clodagh